T0192954

DEVELOPING PHYSICIAN LEADERS FOR SUCCESSFUL CLINICAL INTEGRATION

ACHE Management Series Editorial Board

Natalie D. Lamberton, Chairman
The Medical Center of Aurora

Christina R. Campos
Guadalupe County Hospital

Jaquetta B. Clemons, DrPH
Christus Spohn Health System

David A. Disbrow, FACHE
University of Cincinnati

Scott A. Haraty, FACHE
North Chicago VA Medical Center

Virginia Larson, FACHE
Albert Lea Medical Center–Mayo Health System

Paul A. Milton, FACHE
Ellis Hospital

Greg Napps, FACHE
Culpeper Regional Hospital

CPT Joseph L. Sanchez Jr.
US Air Force

Megan Schmidt, FACHE
Select Specialty Hospital

Arthur S. Shorr, FACHE
Arthur S. Shorr & Associates Inc.

Janet C. Sternberg, FACHE
Huron Medical Center

DEVELOPING PHYSICIAN LEADERS FOR SUCCESSFUL CLINICAL INTEGRATION

Carson F. Dye and Jacque J. Sokolov

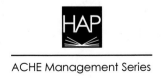

ACHE Management Series

Your board, staff, or clients may also benefit from this book's insight. For more information on quantity discounts, contact the Health Administration Press Marketing Manager at (312) 424–9470.

This publication is intended to provide accurate and authoritative information in regard to the subject matter covered. It is sold, or otherwise provided, with the understanding that the publisher is not engaged in rendering professional services. If professional advice or other expert assistance is required, the services of a competent professional should be sought.

The statements and opinions contained in this book are strictly those of the authors and do not represent the official positions of the American College of Healthcare Executives or the Foundation of the American College of Healthcare Executives.

Copyright © 2013 by the Foundation of the American College of Healthcare Executives. Printed in the United States of America. All rights reserved. This book or parts thereof may not be reproduced in any form without written permission of the publisher.

Reprinted March 2019

Library of Congress Cataloging-in-Publication Data

Dye, Carson F.
  Developing physician leaders for successful clinical integration / by Carson F. Dye and Jacque J. Sokolov.
    pages cm
  ISBN 978-1-56793-554-7 (alk. paper)
  1. Physician executives. 2. Hospitals—Administration. 3. Leadership. I. Sokolov, Jacque J. II. Title.
  RA972.D94 2013
  362.17'2—dc23
                    2012036073

The paper used in this publication meets the minimum requirements of American National Standard for Information Sciences—Permanence of Paper for Printed Library Materials, ANSI Z39.48-1984. ∞ ™

Acquisitions editor: Janet Davis; Project manager: Amy Carlton; Cover designer: Marisa Jackson; Layout: Virginia Byrne

Found an error or a typo? We want to know! Please e-mail it to hapbooks@ache.org, and put "Book Error" in the subject line.

For photocopying and copyright information, please contact Copyright Clearance Center at www.copyright.com or at (978) 750–8400.

Health Administration Press
A division of the Foundation of the American
   College of Healthcare Executives
One North Franklin Street, Suite 1700
Chicago, IL 60606–3529
(312) 424–2800

For my family
—Carson F. Dye

To my loving family, Mitzi, Mariel Francesca, and Ariana Isabel, and to the previous generation of healthcare executives, both physicians and nonphysicians, whose shoulders I stand on
—Jacque J. Sokolov

Contents

Foreword

Today, more than at any time in American history, healthcare is at a crossroads with respect to its future and sustainability. The Patient Protection and Affordable Care Act (ACA) of 2010 is a game changer that will require all healthcare providers to rethink traditional strategies and approaches to operational management and to reinvent the delivery of healthcare in these unpredictable and turbulent times to survive.

Carson Dye and Jacque Sokolov, MD, through their book *Developing Physician Leaders for Successful Clinical Integration,* provide the healthcare executive with a roadmap to navigate these new waters by integrating physicians into the very fabric of the organization. With this integration, the influence of physicians can be real and meaningful and can ensure that physicians take ownership and pride in their healthcare delivery setting and do not simply respond as "renters." This book will help healthcare executives determine their readiness for accepting physician leadership and understand the value physicians bring to new roles within healthcare management.

More than ever before, the traditional approaches to cost management, patient safety, quality improvement, and the patient experience—all affecting pay for performance—require a divergent direction that brings physicians into true partnership. Giving physicians leadership opportunities helps to set the stage for their input into governance, strategy, policy development, management, and significant engagement in operations, all affecting how we do business in these undefined times. If our goal is to be ready for whatever comes our way regarding healthcare reform, we must be prepared to engage physicians in meaningful leadership positions and develop them accordingly.

Transition and ambiguity are our collective futures; one size does not fit all. And yet we must create organizational values that are inclusive and nimble and acknowledge we are on this journey together—together we succeed or fail. By embracing true physician leadership we can build a culture of collaboration like never before for the benefit of the patients and community we collectively serve.

Steven A. Fellows, FACHE
Executive Vice President and Chief Operating Officer
Cottage Health System
Santa Barbara, California

My career journey started in high school in Tipp City, Ohio, when I decided to make premed my college major. This decision was a result of two major influences in my life—sports and my family physician. This physician served as the team physician for the high-school basketball team, and seeing him in these two roles made me want to be just like him. His desire and interest in helping people and giving back to his community was truly remarkable.

Being involved in sports also helped me understand and appreciate the need for a team in order to win. In team sports, individual success has minimal impact on the ultimate goal, which is to win a game or a championship.

After attending Valparaiso University on a basketball scholarship, I was fortunate to be accepted to The Ohio State University Medical School. From there I was chosen to be a resident in the family practice residency at Miami Valley Hospital in Dayton, Ohio. Following residency, I joined a two-man family practice group in my hometown. My family's physician, my role model, had been a partner in this practice. Unfortunately, he had died two years earlier because of a progressive neurological degenerative disease. Starting my career as a practicing physician by replacing the man who had been my role model was deeply meaningful to me.

I practiced clinical medicine for 17 years, including serving as a team physician for my old high school. My physician executive duties began when I was elected chief of staff at Upper Valley Medical Center at the age of 38. I felt ill prepared for this role, and, like many physician leaders, I jumped in and learned—sometimes the hard way—by experience. My biggest lesson was that getting other viewpoints and opinions is helpful in difficult situations. I also learned that the clinical staff members could exert a strong influence on each other that was sometimes more effective than top-down decisions.

The CEO at the time recognized that physicians had little to no leadership training. He funded my attendance at seminars at the American College of Physician Executives. I found these meetings exciting, interesting, and thought-provoking, and I began to think I could have a greater impact on healthcare as a physician executive than I had as a practicing physician.

I became the medical director of the hospital's employed primary care group (after selling our practice to the hospital) in 1994, and became its first chief medical officer (CMO) in 1997. I was extremely fortunate to be given responsibilities in pharmacy and home health, which were beyond the traditional duties of the CMO or vice president of medical affairs (VPMA). From this experience, I learned about operational planning and the financial side of medicine. Most important, the CMO position gave me a seat at the table with the other senior executives. My opinion was valued and taken into account when the nonphysician CEO made decisions, and I realized that being asked for input *before* the decision had already been made was important to me.

I left my organization in 2000 to become medical director at East Jefferson General Hospital (EJGH) in Metairie, Louisiana, a suburb of New Orleans. I intended to be there two or three years and move on, but in August 2002 I was chosen as interim CEO. At that time, one board member made a statement that would stay with me forever: "We, the board, have one employee—you." That statement quickly put things into perspective and made me realize that moving into the CEO position meant moving into new territory and vast responsibilities.

I am often asked if my long-term goal was to become a CEO. The answer is no. At the same time, as my career evolved and moved forward, I became convinced that physician leadership was vital for successful healthcare organizations. I do not think that every organization needs to be led by a physician; I do think that successful organizations need to have engaged physician leadership. I also believe that high-performing organizations have moved beyond thinking of physician leaders only in the traditional VPMA or CMO roles. As healthcare is rapidly evolving, physicians need to be directly involved with strategic and operational discussions and decisions. The life of a practicing physician is also changing dramatically. Not including physicians in key decisions is shortsighted and foolhardy.

Through basketball, I learned that building a strong team means placing less emphasis on individual accomplishments, much as physicians must learn to trade some of their independence for the greater goal. And based on my own career, I believe management and leadership educational programs are valuable, but they must be combined with real-life experiences for successful physician leadership. Carson Dye and Jacque Sokolov have written a book that echoes my conclusions about healthcare organizations and physician leaders. But their book has also allowed me to make new connections and develop new insights. In these pages you will find both great strategy and practical suggestions to enhance the role physicians play in leadership. Even those who believe they already "get" physician leadership will benefit from reading this book.

Mark J. Peters, MD
President and CEO
East Jefferson General Hospital
Metairie, Louisiana

Preface

The push toward population health, outcomes-based reimbursement, and greater accountability necessitate that hospitals groom physician leaders. How good a job do we do in training physician leaders? Do we pick out potential candidates and groom them?

—*David Nash, MD, dean, School of Population Health, Thomas Jefferson University (Weinstock 2011)*

A CLEAR LOOK AT A CONTROVERSIAL TOPIC

We present this book to you with great respect and humility. This topic is often loaded with strong emotion and passion. So many divergent views exist on the topic, some causing great divisiveness. We have engaged in many spirited and, at times, heated dialogues with both physicians and nonphysicians in the development of this book. We hope to present a neutral but strong clarion call for an enhancement of our industry's efforts to prepare and deploy more physician leaders.

We do not wish to be divisive, but we do make many evaluative and prescriptive comments in the book. We share these general thoughts with you the reader in hopes that you will understand our thoughts and approach as we crafted this text.

These beliefs and viewpoints shaped our thoughts as we wrote.

A TSUNAMI OF CHANGES MEANS DEMAND FOR PHYSICIAN LEADERS

We see more significant change in healthcare in the United States now than at any other time in history. Although this statement could be hyperbolic, we do believe it. We think the entire shape and form of healthcare delivery will be substantially changed in the next ten years. Although most of the changes are being driven by economic reasons, much of the transformation—and we do mean *transformation*—will be physician-centric.

We believe that quality has finally taken a front seat in the healthcare industry, and we contend this is a good thing. We see two drivers for this change: several Institute of Medicine reports (2012, 2006a, 2006b, 2003a, 2003b, 2001, 1999) and the determination by payers—and consumers—that they want more value for their dollar.

Because of this and several other factors, we strongly feel that there will be an enormous demand for more physician leaders who are better trained, better educated, and better prepared to lead.

CLINICAL INTEGRATION

Healthcare has been on a path to clinical integration for decades, but the market forces driving us in that direction—fueled by economics, reform, and patient and payer preference—are stronger than ever. Back in the day—the 1980s and 1990s, if you remember that particular part of "way back when"—the talk was about "integrated delivery systems" and "pay-for-performance" programs. Now that emphasis on providers working together on the value of the services they provide has matured. Now not just the means of delivering care services must be integrated, but the services themselves must be coordinated toward a result, not an amount required to make a profit. Now providers must be paid not just for meeting evidence-based care guidelines but for providing value for the money that payers and plan sponsors spend. And we must strongly suggest this change is not just Capitation 2.0. We feel that capitation was an economically driven concept, while this new clinical integration world is physician-centric.

That distinction means physicians and hospitals—and all the ancillaries, devices, and diagnostics they have at their disposal—must be better aligned across broad clinical categories if providers hope to offer the type of value-based care that payers and patients demand. And that means physicians must step up and assume leadership roles in healthcare organizations that were heretofore considered the exclusive purview of career business executives. Physicians' hard-earned understanding of what works and what does not—and at what cost—from a clinical patient care perspective is the driver of the new normal in healthcare. *Meaningful clinical integration* is not just a catchphrase or a buzzword. It is a roadmap to survival.

PHYSICIAN LEADERSHIP DEVELOPMENT EFFORTS ARE RAPIDLY CHANGING

We feel that even the best efforts at creating physician leadership development programs in the past were poor compared to the better-focused approaches that are beginning to be used today. We believe differences exist between management and leadership positions, which explains part of the problem with physician leadership development activities. We do not feel, as some do, that management is "bad" and leadership is "good." Rather, some positions involve mostly management, some involve mostly leadership, and some are a blend of both. We feel these considerations are important in physician leadership development, and we highlight these differences throughout the book. We feel as well that current efforts are beginning to recognize the unique skills that physicians bring to both disciplines (management and leadership) and the critical role those skills play in creating and managing a clinically integrated organization.

JUMPING IN

We recognize that among the challenges and difficulties in writing this book is the fact that organizations are at many different stages in physician leadership and involvement. Some are advanced; some are just beginning. Some still have traditional medical staff models, while others have scrapped those models entirely. Some have all employed physicians and some have few. Some focus on grooming physician leaders rather than physician managers, and some recognize that both are crucial to the future functioning of a healthcare organization.

Moreover, we recognize the many divergent views on this topic. Engaging physicians in the development and management of a clinically integrated healthcare organization is fundamental to the success of every provider organization in this country. But not everyone is ready to embrace tomorrow and leave yesterday behind. We have tried to focus on the future, on the critical need to bring physicians into the leadership loop. We ask you, the reader, to approach our material with an open mind and a seeking spirit. We do not have all the answers. But we feel this book will serve as a good guide for exploration.

Ultimately, we hope to bring value to our industry.

Thank you for reading.

—*Carson Dye and Jacque Sokolov*

Acknowledgments

My executive search work lets me meet many great leaders and learn about many great organizations. In some respects, if I just listen and act as a sponge, I pick up hundreds of books' worth of excellence and impact leadership. I have interviewed and visited with so many physician leaders and executives over the years and have been truly enriched by their visions, accomplishments, thoughts, and experiences. In reality, I owe acknowledgments to far more people than I could list. So, first of all, to those who are not listed but from whom I have gained in knowledge and perspective, thanks.

Second, I want to acknowledge several doctors who have touched me along the way and given me insight and thoughts that have helped stimulate many of the ideas in this book. To begin with, I must lift my hat high for Dr. Greg Taylor. Greg and I taught an American College of Healthcare Executives course on physician leadership for several years in the 1990s, and he was a great partner. Like many great physician leaders, Greg has moved higher in his own physician leadership career and is a chief operating officer and a Baldrige examiner as well as a great friend. I make special note of my friend and fellow Health Administration Press (HAP) author, Dr. Ken Cohn. Ken does great work in helping others work collaboratively with physicians; he is constantly adding to our insight about physician leadership. Dr. Scott Ransom, CEO of the University of North Texas Health Science Center, has been a great friend and colleague over the years. A former president of the American College of Physician Executives, former chief medical officer and chief quality officer, and a former executive search colleague, Scott has given me much to think about as I have pondered the leadership roles of physicians in healthcare. Dr. Mark Peters, who was so gracious to write one of our forewords, is owed a note of thanks as well. I have observed and learned from his leadership over the years. I also thank the writer of our other foreword, Steve Fellows, another HAP author and an individual who has a great record of positive relationships with physicians. He truly respects the role physicians can play in leadership. It has also been an honor to get to know Dr. Mark Laney and gain from his viewpoints on physician leadership. I also owe thanks to a number of physicians with whom I have interacted at various meetings of The Healthcare Roundtable and elsewhere. While I hate to overlook anyone, I would include in that list Drs. Steve Markovich, Dave Kapaska, Imran Andrabi, John Byrnes, Kathy Forbes, David Tam, Cliff Devenny, Tom McGann, Courtenay Beebe, Dee Russell, John Fortney, John Kosanovich, Stacy Goldsholl, Ronnie Brownsworth, Robin Ledyard, Bill VanNess, and John Paris. These physicians likely do not know the influence they have had on my thinking about physician leadership, but my exposure to them has enriched me. I consider them to be great physician leader role models and could easily see them entering into a physician leadership hall of fame. Several individuals gave great insight into several of our chapters. They include Dr. John Redding, Blue Consulting, one of the nation's experts in clinical integration. John served as a contributor in several of the more complex areas of the book. Frank Sheeder from DLA Piper and Jeff Kapp from Jones Day, two great healthcare attorneys, gave assistance on some of the finer legal points. I am also very appreciative to Dr. Lee Hammerling with ProMedica in Toledo. A friend for many years, he has given me interesting insight into transitions that physicians make as they move into leadership. He also helped provide one of our great case studies. Also graciously providing case studies were Dr. Mark Laney, president and CEO of Heartland Health; Martha Davis, director, Organizational Consulting; Laird Covey, president, Central Maine Medical Center; and David Frum, president, Bridgton Hospital and Rumford Hospital. I truly appreciate the willingness of these leaders to share their successes so openly.

Thanks go as well to Mike Covert, with whom I have worked, learned, and taught for years. I have also gained from working with people such as Gene Miyamoto, Mark Hannahan, Kam Sigafoos, and Bill Sanger, four individuals who had a true fondness and respect for physicians and have had great success as a result. As I reflect about what makes leaders great, I strongly believe that we grow through osmosis from others. Whether through formal mentoring, role modeling, or simple observations, I have had the great fortune to be around many strong leaders, physician and nonphysician, who knew how to weave physicians into the equation of organizational leadership. I would also recognize Russell Jackson, who helped Jacque and me so much on this book, and Jacque's worthy assistant, Sue Pearce, who kept us all together. I am thankful for my daughter, Emily, who helped design the creative and helpful conceptual selection model used in this book.

This book marks 20 years and eight books with Health Administration Press (HAP). I cannot say it more clearly: HAP is a great asset to our field. Janet Davis has been a great pleasure to work with, and I salute her enthusiasm and support. Behind the scenes, she helps to bring us great offerings in healthcare knowledge. I am also grateful for the excitement that Amy Carlton took in editing this book; her insight was quite helpful. It is quite fulfilling when your editor gets excited about your work—she did, and this inspired me further. Readers, if you ever have the chance, stop and see the HAP staff and thank them for their service to us.

As I conclude, I reach the point of talking about Jacque. Dr. Jacque Sokolov, my coauthor, deserves great recognition. What an honor it has been to work with him. He is such a great futuristic thinker, yet he is so grounded in the reality of today's leadership challenges. His experiences cross many types of organizations, and this adds to his creative insight. I was stretched by him and gained much from our interactions.

My final acknowledgment—to those physicians who are already in leadership roles, and to those who will be moving into them, thanks for your service. You truly do make a difference.

—*Carson F. Dye, FACHE*

The next generation of clinical integration and the resulting enhanced physician leadership opportunities represent a key tipping point for organizational physician involvement at the governance, management, and operating levels. From an editorial and coauthor perspective, permit me to acknowledge my colleague and friend, Carson Dye, who represents all things good that a coauthor can be—knowledgeable, patient, and insightful.

To acknowledge everyone who has contributed to my professional development both in the physician and nonphysician executive world would require another entire book, but you know who you are, and you know how limitless my gratitude is to all of you.

Academically, professors, mentors, and colleagues from the University of Southern California, the USC School of Medicine, the Mayo Clinic, and the University of Texas Southwestern Medical School all provided an unparalleled clinical foundation for me to build on. The professional associations, including The Society for Medical Administrators, the Medical Administrators Conference, the Duke Private Sector Conference, the Washington Business Group on Health, and many more gave me additional insights with giants in the industry. I stand on the shoulders of such leaders as Drs. James Willerson, Edward Rosenow, Jr., Ralph Snyderman, Richard Janeway, Michael Johns, Paul Torrens, Robert Tranquada, Edward Zapanta, George Haidet, and too many others to count.

I must acknowledge the guidance of three exceptional people, first of whom is my father, a remarkable clinician, human being, and dedicated provider of care to his patients for more than 40 years. He had the confidence in me to encourage the nontraditional pathway of being a physician executive before the term "physician executive" even existed. In addition, I would be significantly remiss if I did not thank Howard Allen, the chairman, president, and CEO of Southern California Edison Company (SCE), for providing me with my first physician executive leadership position. In addition to Mr. Allen, many SCE board members, officers, and managers supported many challenging efforts during many challenging times. Mr. Allen, in particular, threw his formidable intellect, influence, and courage behind what turned out to be prescient difficult corporate decisions that many other CEOs in other industries failed to understand for decades and sometimes not until their companies were in Chapter 11. Additionally, I wish to thank David Jones, Sr., chairman, president, CEO, and cofounder of Humana, who provided me with the wisdom that success is something you earn every day, and exceptional times call for exceptional creativity and nontraditional solutions. I stand on their shoulders as well.

Some names stand out, especially in the context of this book. Michael Treacy, Stephen Bennett, Ted Schwab, Chris Schaefer, Mitzi Krockover, MD, David Liff, Ron Anderson, Michael Karlin, and Rita and Steve Moya all have contributed to the success of SSB Solutions, Inc., which has provided many of the case studies cited in this book. One of those case studies involves Bob Meyer, the extremely able CEO and president of Phoenix Children's Hospital. His efforts to improve the quality of care at his institution by comprehensive integration of all clinical services being delivered there provide an example every health system executive can look to for guidance in structuring tomorrow's enterprisewide quality initiatives. As well, I must point out the exceptional work of Todd Sorensen, MD, the dedicated CEO and president of Regional West Medical Center and Health Services. Todd, and his father before him, focused on providing exceptional healthcare in a difficult geographic locale. Todd took a near-moribund program that was the center of Scottsbluff, Nebraska's healthcare and economic world and brought it back to life. He has been a valued colleague and inspiration for the past ten years. He is a great example of physician leadership that makes a difference in the real world and as an indispensable community resource.

Indeed, over the years it has been a pleasure working with the ongoing efforts of industry-leading organizations like the American Medical Association, American Hospital Association, the American Medical Group Association, the Voluntary Hospital Association, the Medical Group Management Association, the American College of Physician Executives, the American Association of Medical Colleges, the National Fund for Medical Education, the White House Health Project, the Alliance for Healthcare Reform, the American Board of Medical Quality, and many more organizations for their constant championing of meaningful reforms in healthcare policy and patient advocacy. In addition, I owe a continuing debt of professional gratitude to the dedicated, forward-thinking executives at the healthcare organizations where I am lucky enough to have ongoing relationships: Hospira; MedCath Corp.; the National Health Foundation; SSB Solutions, Inc.; Healthcare Community Development Group, LLC; and My Health Direct Inc., just to name a few.

I'm proud to profess my sincere admiration for and thanks to the editorial staff at HAP, whose guidance in assembling our executive ideas has proved invaluable. I must note as well my thanks to Russell Jackson, who helps me put my ideas into words, and Sue Pearce, who is invaluable in virtually every aspect of my professional life.

And finally, of course, I wish to especially thank my wife, Dr. Mitzi Krockover. Mitzi, as the founding director of the Iris Cantor–UCLA Women's Health Center and Humana corporate vice president, women's health and e-health, has always been an exemplary influence in professionalism, compassion, and the greater good for her patients and beneficiaries. I would not be a dad if I did not thank, with enormous pride, my daughters Mariel and Ariana, who teach me things each day that make my life more complete and personally joyful.

—*Jacque J. Sokolov, MD*

Introduction

How critical is physician leadership to a healthcare organization's strategy?

It was important to have physician leaders throughout the enterprise.... It creates accountability, and it is a model that gives physicians an equal share of authority and responsibility.

> —*R. Bruce Wellman, MD, chief executive officer of the Carle Physician Group, during a session at the Healthcare Financial Management Association's 2011 Annual National Institute*

Physicians need to be in leadership roles. It's more than just having physicians on the board.

> —*Mary C. Reed, vice president of Gateway Health, part of the Gateway Group in Cleveland*

Physician involvement in health-system decision making and their support of health-system initiatives can be critical to a health system's success.

> —*R. J. Solomon, 2004*

Once we got physicians more heavily involved on an ongoing basis in our board committees and provided routine mechanisms for them to give us input into management decision making, we started to see a reduction in physician complaints, increased physician engagement, attendance at medical staff meetings, and better interaction between our physicians and hospital staff.

> —*Midwest hospital CEO, October 2011*

Physician leadership, enhanced quality, improved value for patients, cost reduction, evidence-based practice, organizational efficiencies, clinical integration, accountable care organizations, physician involvement, value-based payment, physician leadership. It starts and ends with physician leadership.

This book is designed to challenge leaders in the healthcare industry to rise to a higher level of action in developing and involving physician leaders. This call for action is based on the premise that physicians must be far more involved in crafting strategy and in executive, managerial, and organizational decision making for healthcare organizations to be more effective. With the help of the practical suggestions presented in the chapters ahead, organizations can identify, involve, develop, and facilitate the clinical integration of extraordinary physician leaders. We intend this book to serve as a clarion call to intensify the efforts of physician leadership development in the healthcare industry.

OVERVIEW

Multiple factors (see "Factors Driving Greater Interest in Physician Leadership") have converged to create a major nexus that will make physician leadership of health enterprises more vital than ever.

Factors Driving Greater Interest in Physician Leadership

- Significant changes in the healthcare delivery system
- Greater emphasis on quality and patient safety
- Reimbursement mechanisms now paying for value, not volume
- Growth of population health management
- Movement from acute care to ambulatory and home care
- Different styles in the practice of medicine
- Newer physicians expecting more input
- Movement toward the employment of physicians by health systems and corporations
- Clinical integration

Few will dispute that the traditional medical staff model is broken. The proliferation of employed physicians and the decline of independent practitioners have made the traditional elected medical staff leadership prototype look like a twentieth-century relic. Moreover, the fact that few, if any, primary care physicians are physically present at acute care facilities—in addition to the rapid growth of inpatient hospitalists—means the physician collective is now split into parts. Not enough physicians are prepared to take management and leadership positions. A new breed of physicians, whose goal is to practice medicine without being involved in committee work or medical staff–elected leadership roles, has surfaced. Unlike their predecessors, many physicians today may also expect compensation for time spent on leadership.

Consider as well for a moment the impact physicians have on the activities of the healthcare enterprise. The physician's order creates every activity involved in healthcare. This drives costs. Healthcare costs are growing at an unsustainable rate and are a major source of future unfunded liabilities in the United States. In addition, the cost shifting that has been done inside healthcare for the past 50 years will soon end, and reimbursement will place a greater emphasis on performance and risk bearing by providers. All of these changes must occur through the redirection of physicians.

The bottom line of this current state of affairs is that healthcare enterprises will be strongly focused on reducing costs, transforming the way care is delivered, increasing preventive care, improving quality, creating larger and more efficient care delivery entities, reducing unnecessary utilization, integrating community health into the system, and placing a greater emphasis on wellness (see Exhibit 1). Physicians *must* lead these efforts.

A comment on other healthcare providers is appropriate here. This book *does not ignore* the many types of trained health professionals who take care of patients.

Exhibit 1: Clinical Care/Reimbursement Models Leading to More Physician–Hospital Integration

The Healthcare Ecosystem
Increasingly aligned interests and integration opportunities

Pressures on Physicians
- Declining payer reimbursement/self-pay % grows
- Declining revenue from ancillaries
- PCP shortages
- Specialist shortages
- Recruiting challenges
- Increased practice overhead
- Growing regulatory requirements

Physician Community ⟳ Hospitals

Pressures on Hospitals
- Pluralistic medical staff
- Declining payer reimbursement/self-pay % grows
- Increased competition from specialty hospitals
- Physician-sponsored OP competition
- Rise of P4P programs
- Increased consumer expectations
- Regulatory demands

Hospital-Sponsored Medical Group
MD/DO Employment
Comanagement
PSHP/PSHN/ACO/Medical Home

Nurses, nurse practitioners, physician assistants, pharmacists, physical therapists, occupational therapists, radiologic technicians, medical technologists, and countless others certainly play essential roles in the care of patients. These dedicated caregivers clearly will hold larger and greater roles in the future. But the physician has historically led the care teams—and the physician is front and center in the majority of changes that will occur in the coming years. We write this book with the utmost respect to all health professionals, but our primary objective is to target the physician and the need for leadership roles for physicians in the industry.

THE TARGET AUDIENCE FOR THIS BOOK

This book will hit home with healthcare leaders who identify with any of the following viewpoints:

- "I strongly believe that physicians need to take a more active leadership role in my healthcare organization."
- "Over time, these physician leadership roles will include physicians serving in full-time executive and managerial roles—and not just as traditional chief medical officers or vice presidents of medical affairs. That means many of these physicians will step out of their clinical roles and serve exclusively in full-time administrative leadership positions."
- "An increasing number of physicians will soon move into chief operating officer and chief executive officer positions."
- "Our field is in a process of many shifts for physicians:
  - from an era of independent physicians practicing in their own private corporations to models with physicians functioning as employees of larger corporate entities;
  - from primary care physicians working in and around acute care facilities to many physicians never setting foot inside those types of facilities;
  - from generalists to even more highly specialized clinicians, including hospitalists;
  - from the traditional medical staff model of governance to a corporate practice of medicine; and
  - from physicians serving in advisory capacities to executive management to physicians actually being executive managers."
- "These factors and many others are having a massive impact upon my organization, and physician leadership is needed to help guide us through the changes."

- "I am now persuaded that I need to take significant efforts to grow and develop more physician leaders and to enhance physician involvement in the leadership of my organization. I want to know where to begin."

Key questions for consideration:

- How are physician leaders identified?
- How does physician leadership development most effectively get integrated into the fabric of an organization?
- Assuming that one of the key methods of developing leaders is to involve them in leadership matters, how should physicians be involved in policy setting, strategy deliberation, and decision making in a healthcare organization?
- What does the term *physician leadership* mean? What does it mean for an organization to be *physician led*?
- What type of leadership education should be provided to physicians who are formal and informal leaders within the collective physician community? What are the more effective approaches to a physician leadership development program?

TWO POSSIBLY CONTROVERSIAL THOUGHTS

First, although the book will not address this issue in a provocative manner, the authors feel that most efforts at physician leadership development have been dismal and have produced limited results, including the following:

- Although many dollars have been spent on educating physicians in leadership skills, most programs have been haphazard, not woven into any type of organizational strategy, and rarely well coordinated (e.g., attendance at conferences sponsored by large educational organizations whose programs have little local application once physician leaders return home).
- Many physician leadership development programs are left to a speaker at the occasional quarterly medical staff meeting or to external programs where a few key physicians are sent (perhaps in hopes that attending just a few days of meetings will help them return as leaders).
- Even the programs at the larger healthcare organizations with "mini-MBA" programs or physician leadership development "institutes" have not had significant impact.

Second, most efforts at developing physician leaders rarely take the final step of involving them in full-fledged leadership of the healthcare enterprise. *Asking physician leaders for input* on strategy and decision making is not the same as *involving them* in these processes and keeping them at the table throughout the execution and implementation stages (see "Differences Between Involvement and Input").

Differences Between Involvement and Input

Involvement	Input
Physicians are always at decision-making meetings	Physicians are sometimes invited
Physicians are viewed as partners	Physicians are viewed as tokens
Executive leadership sees physicians as aligned	Executive leadership seeks alignment from physicians
Physician involvement is ongoing	Physician input is sporadic
Physicians remain in the process	Physicians are occasional players
Seeing physicians at the table is common	Seeing physicians at the table is rare

Some healthcare leaders may *not* want to fully involve physicians in this manner. While they may be willing to provide physicians with some level of input, they prefer that the ultimate decision-making authority rest with them. As one CEO commented, "Their [physicians'] job is to care for patients; my job is to run the hospital." Another executive said, "Doctors are simply not trained in business—and they should keep their noses out of business decisions." This dynamic contributes to the mistrust that exists in many organizations and directly affects physician leadership development.

SOME THOUGHTS ON PHYSICIAN LEADERSHIP DEVELOPMENT

Developing physician leadership is an expensive proposition, both financially and in terms of the time commitment required by physicians and the health system. Yet to do it well, organizations must be prepared to make exactly that commitment.

Today, an unprecedented number of ways exist to educate physician leaders, and organizations need help and direction in sorting these out.

Future gains in quality and in health system and physician alignment will be made only through a greatly increased amount of physician involvement—including physician CEOs. Beyond the question of physician CEOs, healthcare needs physician input, counsel, participation, collaboration, and involvement at many different levels.

The following themes are important for strong physician leadership development (see Exhibit 2):

How physician leaders are identified. Organizations must formally and informally identify leaders within the physician community for further development. This process should be similar to strategic planning.

How healthcare organizations meaningfully involve physicians in strategy development, policy setting, and decision making. Organizations must do a better job of providing physicians with true authority in the management of the enterprise (which is the result of true integration and alignment). For optimal physician leadership development, physician leaders must have high levels of involvement

Exhibit 2: The Physician Leadership and Involvement Model

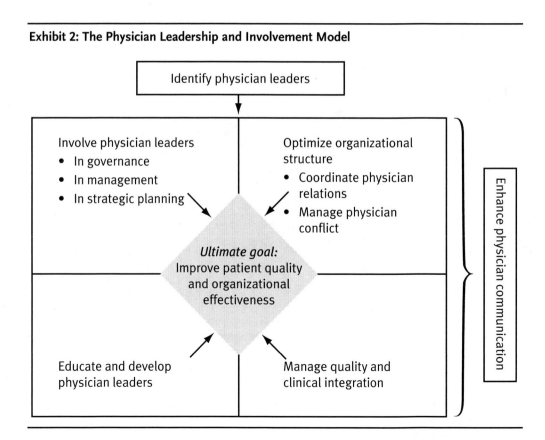

in governance, management, and strategy development and must be appointed to formal positions of authority in the healthcare organization.

How physicians are developed as leaders. Organizations must use contemporary leadership development approaches to adequately develop physician leaders. Effective physician leadership development goes beyond educational program curriculum design to place emphasis on active learning, developmental exercises, and experiential learning (on-the-job training).

The clinical integration of physicians. Organizations must take steps toward clinical integration and manage it in sync with physician leadership development.

The role of physicians in leading quality. Clearly, the future healthcare organizations that will be most effective will be those that lead in quality. Physician leadership will be integral in ensuring that quality takes a front seat in the organization's priorities (see Exhibit 3).

Exhibit 3: Example of Aligned Clinical and Business Vision

Components are integrated into shared and aligned vision for hospital services and the hospital-sponsored medical group

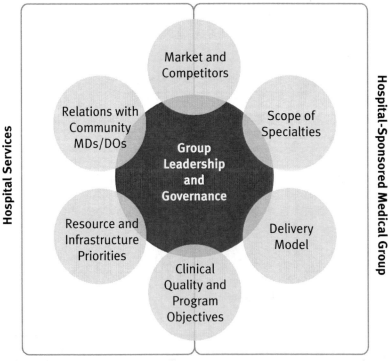

ORGANIZATION OF THIS BOOK

Chapter 1 opens with a discussion on the special nature of physicians—their role in the healthcare enterprise and their impact on quality, costs, and outcomes. It gives a deep understanding of the nature of physician education and differences from other educational avenues, and it is intended to provide readers a foundation for better understanding physicians as they begin to address leadership and involvement matters.

Chapter 2 introduces and explores what it means for an organization to be physician led. Further discussion on the nature of physician-led organizations and implications for organizations that increase the amount of physician involvement in leadership is provided.

Chapter 3 presents a summary of opinions from a group of physician leaders and is designed to provide a quick snapshot of what we have traditionally done in our industry with physician leadership.

Part II, containing Chapters 4 through 8, provides a guide to some of the critical first steps that most organizations take in enhancing physician leadership. While some organizations will have already implemented many of these concepts and suggestions, others will only be beginning. Chapter 4 provides an innovative look at how to identify physician leaders. The concepts presented can be used to start a leadership development program and can also help in establishing a physician leadership selection process. Chapter 5 draws attention to an important distinction that is often overlooked—the difference between management positions and leadership positions. This distinction is important as more physicians join both management and leadership ranks. Chapter 6 looks at the vice president of medical affairs position and how it is undergoing a major transition. Chapter 7 discusses some of the more important issues involved as physicians begin to transition into either part-time or full-time leadership and management roles. Finally, Chapter 8 provides a primer on physician relations and gives an outline of some of the organizational cornerstones that need to be in place to move forward with physician leadership development.

Part III identifies many of the significant changes that are about to affect our industry and require stronger physician involvement and leadership. Chapter 9 gives an overview of some of the industry changes that will increase demand for profound clinical integration. Chapter 10 provides a how-to approach to building a clinically integrated organization. Chapter 11 looks at an enterprise quality plan and shows detailed steps and suggestions on how to build one. Chapter 12, a useful hands-on guide, gives an in-depth approach to assessing and selecting physician leaders. Chapter 13 gives a brief overview of how to educate physician leaders.

Chapter 14 provides some specific case samples that demonstrate that enhancing physician leadership goes beyond developing a simple educational curriculum. Chapter 15 provides contemporary thoughts and research that explains why senior leaders often derail in their leadership career—a matter that is particularly troublesome with physician leaders. Finally, Chapter 16 serves as an epilogue from the authors—a brief snapshot of what the future might look like.

Appendixes provide specific tools that can be used to evaluate an organization's readiness for clinical integration as well as two sample letters detailing what leaders should tell physicians who are thinking of moving into leadership roles. Two physician candidate evaluation tools are also provided to help organizations think about how they might evaluate physician leaders. Finally, an assessment tool is provided for readers who want to jump-start their plan to build more effective physician leadership development programs.

Although much of our focus in this book will be on employed full-time and part-time physician leaders, we also realize that, for many organizations, the first steps in growing physician leadership will be launched in organizations with physicians who are still independent practitioners. Our crystal ball suggests that, ultimately, most if not all physicians will be employed by some type of larger healthcare organization, and as a result, the number of full-time employed physician leaders will grow.

CONCLUSION

Judging from the calls at healthcare conferences around the country for increased and more effective physician leadership and the input that we have received from many healthcare leaders, a tidal wave of interest in improving physician leadership has hit the healthcare industry. This book will become a hornbook for those with their hands on the levers of change.

Thoughts for Consideration

To what extent has your organization prepared physician leaders?

How supportive are your organization's senior leaders (board and management) of the precepts included in this introductory chapter?

SUGGESTED READING

Fairchild, D. G., E. M. Benjamin, D. R. Gifford, and S. J. Huot. 2004. "Physician Leadership: Enhancing the Career Development of Academic Physician Administrators and Leaders." *Academic Medicine* 79 (3): 214–18.

Serio, C. D., and T. Epperly. 2006. "Physician Leadership: A New Model for a New Generation: Today's Leaders Need More Than Vision and a High IQ." *Family Practice Management* 13 (2): 51–54.

Zuckerman, H. S., D. W. Hilberman, R. M. Andersen, L. R. Burns, J. A. Alexander, and P. Torrens. 1998. "Physicians and Organizations: Strange Bedfellows or a Marriage Made in Heaven?" *Frontiers of Health Services Management* 14 (3): 3–34.

Note: The authors have made their best efforts to provide information that is complete and accurate at the time of publication. However, all articles and any forms, checklists, guidelines, and materials are for general information only and should not be used or referred to as primary legal sources nor construed as establishing medical standards of care. They are intended as resources to be selectively used and always adapted—with the advice of the organization's attorney—to meet state, local, and individual organizations' needs or requirements. This book is distributed with the understanding that neither the authors nor the publisher is engaged in rendering legal services or medical advice.

Part I

MAKING THE CASE FOR GREATER PHYSICIAN INVOLVEMENT

CHAPTER 1

Physicians

Men who are occupied in the restoration of health to other men, by the joint exertion of skill and humanity, are above all the great of the earth. They even partake of divinity, since to preserve and renew is almost as noble as to create.
—*Voltaire*

God heals and the doctor takes the fees.
—*Benjamin Franklin*

Physicians are a popular topic of conversation. Few people lack opinions about them. Yet few fully understand the nature of physicians' education, their preparation, or the issues they face. Sadly, this is also true of some nonphysician administrators.

Despite being at the core of what happens to patients, physicians are often far from the core of decisions related to how patients are managed. Unfortunately, some healthcare leaders view physicians primarily as widget producers. Physicians are educated in clinical matters; their curriculum does not allow much time for management and leadership training. Having a deep understanding of the nature of physicians is necessary before undertaking any changes to any healthcare system.

Before beginning to build a physician leadership development program, understanding physicians, their typical background, education, and propensities is important. This may seem counterintuitive or obvious to some readers, but it is still important as a foundation for the many considerations proposed throughout this book. This chapter sets the tone for the book with a discussion on the special nature of physicians—their role in the healthcare enterprise; their impact on quality, costs, and outcomes; their seemingly opposite nature to nonphysician administrators; and the critical role they will play in future clinical integration. This chapter asks the reader to gain a foundational understanding of the nature of physician education and its differences from other educational avenues. It respectfully suggests that many nonphysicians do not fully comprehend the role that physicians play in the process of health. Moreover, many do not fully grasp the viewpoints and philosophies of physicians to properly integrate them into organizational decision making. Our hope is that this chapter will draw attention to the need for enhanced physician involvement and leadership.

Questions to ponder at this point:

- Are physicians really any different from any other professionals?
- By using the word *special* in the opening paragraph of this chapter, have we as authors set up artificial barriers?
- Are we according too much deference and reverence to those who are, in fact, really just some of many players on the healthcare stage?

These questions and similar ones can cause heated debate in healthcare circles. However, within the healthcare field, physicians are the drivers. Physicians generate the orders for patient treatments and, as one CEO said, "They are the top of the food chain." The courts and laws and regulations have long spelled out physicians' premier role in the provision of healthcare services. Essentially, under most state laws, little can be done to or for a patient without a physician's order.

Describing physicians can (a) bring up a lot of stereotypes (see the quotes throughout this chapter); (b) be akin to the old tale of the blind men describing an elephant by touch—it depends on the part of the elephant being felt; and (c) result in different assessments depending on whether or not you are a physician—perhaps "you have to be in the club to know the secret handshake." And some understanding may relate to whether you actually respect (or do not respect) physicians.

To what extent are our views of physicians driven by factors such as these? "Doctors are sometimes portrayed as heartless individuals who make too much money and do not care about the patients they are supposed to be treating, or as egomaniacs who like being the center of attention. I do not, and never will, understand either of these descriptions of a physician, and do not understand how we as a society ever got to this point" (Prime Education 2007).

We believe understanding physicians includes knowledge of their educational preparation, a sense of their typical value systems, the contrast between physicians and administrators, awareness of what physicians do, and insight into what physicians are typically like.

To begin, we'll briefly describe the educational preparation of physicians, because this is one of the primary differences that often sets them apart from other professionals.

HOW PHYSICIANS PREPARE: THE EDUCATION PROCESS

The process of selecting a medical school class is complex and intense. American medical schools receive, on average, 31 applications for each place in the entering class, with a range of 2.5 applications for each place among public medical schools to 76 applications among private medical schools.
—*Association of American Medical Colleges, 2012*

> No physician, in so far as he is a physician, considers his own good in what he prescribes, but the good of his patient; for the true physician is also a ruler, having the human body as a subject, and is not a mere money-maker.
> —*Plato*

The education of physicians is typically much longer and more complex than that of any other profession. It entails undergraduate education (such as a degree in biology), medical school, and graduate medical education (a residency and fellowship). Medical school typically takes four years, awards an MD or DO degree, and is followed by three to seven years of specialized residency training and, for some, another one to three years of focused additional training. After completing the required graduate medical education (GME), a physician then applies for a license to practice medicine issued from a state where she plans to practice.

All these years of education led one physician executive to remark, "I was 32 years old before I got my first job."

Board certification, an optional and voluntary process, involves another round of testing. Certification indicates that physicians have been tested on knowledge and skills in a specialty. Currently, 24 specialty boards manage the board certification process, and physicians can be certified in 36 general medical specialties and 88 subspecialty fields. Finally, physicians are required under state laws to take continuing medical education—the CME that some nonphysicians confuse with the also-required GME described previously—to renew their licenses.

> Physicians. Oh, my, what a different breed! And what they say about trying to lead them being like trying to herd cats is so true. Oh, you can't live with them and you can't live without them.
> —*Anonymous hospital CEO, circa 2009*

Changing the Way Physicians Are Educated

Because of the increased complexity of medicine, the move toward more holistic views of medicine, and the segmentation of medicine into specialties, major changes to the manner in which the medical school curriculum is structured are occurring. Readers would benefit from a review of the websites of various medical schools as well as the website of the Association of American Medical Colleges (www.aamc .org) and the Liaison Committee on Medical Education (www.lcme.org) to see how education is changing. Often the goal is greater integration of the "what to do" and the "how to do it in the real world" aspects of medical education.

Indeed, AAMC (2005) notes that thinkers in the medical education realm focus on eight key themes in education reform: technology, financing, workforce development, research and assessment, breaking regulatory barriers in the educational continuum, social accountability, leadership, and trends in healthcare delivery. At a structural level, an AAMC report has called for medical colleges to combine two approaches to future doctor schooling: the "tea bag steeping" approach, which is a time-based model, and "an outcomes-based approach centered on specific learning objectives, with the goal of adapting physicians to the needs of 'users' and strengthening physician 'products' through constant feedback and standardized methods of ensuring safety and quality" (AAMC 2005). The report continues:

> In many medical schools, clinical content has been integrated into the basic science course work offered during the first two years of the educational program. In addition, many schools offer courses in the first two years that focus on various aspects of the doctor–patient relationship, with specific emphasis on taking a history, performing a physical examination, and communicating with patients and patients' families.

The AAMC report added:

> During the past decade, some schools have changed the organization of the third year by creating block rotations. Each of the blocks is composed of several clerkships that students must take in sequence within the block period. More than half of schools [in recent site visits] have adopted this structure. The block structure has been adopted primarily as a means of promoting integration of clinically relevant content across related disciplines (e.g., psychiatry and neurology, pediatrics and obstetrics/gynecology, family medicine and general internal medicine). Several schools have established clerkship blocks that run for three to six months during

the third year. In those schools, the discipline-specific, departmental orientation of individual clerkships has been largely eliminated.

Temple University School of Medicine in Philadelphia, Pennsylvania, recently overhauled its curriculum to better meet the needs of tomorrow's healthcare system. Here is a report from the school's website (2012):

> Doctors are men who prescribe medicines of which they know little, to cure diseases of which they know less, in human beings of whom they know nothing.
> —*Voltaire, circa 1760*

Temple University School of Medicine previously provided a curriculum that was four years in length and culminated in [an] MD degree. It consisted of 158 student instructional weeks, with approximately 25 instructional hours each week in Years 1 and 2 and approximately 45 instructional and patient contact hours each week in Years 3 and 4. Similar to approximately one-third of US medical schools, for several decades, the School of Medicine employed a discipline-based curriculum. In another model, curricula are based on body and organ systems. We believe that such curricula provide better integration of material across basic sciences and between basic and clinical sciences. We have therefore chosen to introduce an Integrated Curriculum [IC].

The curricular content taught in the new IC is similar to the previous curriculum; however, the way in which it is taught has changed. Instead of being divided into a number of courses based in and administered by the academic departments, the IC is now divided into a number of interdisciplinary "blocks." Each block is organized according to body or organ systems and is planned and taught in a coordinated fashion by faculty from a number of basic science and clinical academic departments. As an example, students in the previous curriculum were taught about the normal structure of the body in three different anatomy courses and the normal function of the human body in the physiology and biochemistry courses. Students in the IC are now taught about the cardiovascular system in two "cardiovascular blocks." One block in Year 1 presents in an integrated fashion the relevant anatomy, biochemistry, and physiology. A second block in Year 2 presents the major disease processes (pathology and pathophysiology) and therapeutic options (pharmacology, pathophysiology, medicine, surgery).

The clerkships in Years 3 and 4 are now discipline-based, similar to the previous curriculum, but there are some modifications. The clerkship in neurology has moved from Year 4 to Year 3. Ambulatory medicine in the new, integrated curriculum now receives additional emphasis in Year 3. In Year 4, required clerkships have been added in radiology and critical care medicine. The number of elective clerkships has been reduced from five to four. Teaching strategies now place additional emphasis on the incorporation of basic science principles into clinical medicine.

Identical to the previous curriculum, Temple University School of Medicine's new IC consists of 158 weeks of instruction over four years leading to the MD degree, but without areas of concentration or specialization. Instruction in Years 1 and 2 has been shortened from the previous 75 weeks to 70 weeks. Instruction in Years 3 and 4 has been lengthened from the current 83 weeks to 88 weeks. The Year 3 portion of the curriculum, instead of beginning in July of the third year, now begins in May of the second year and concludes in April of the third year, followed immediately by the Year 4 portion of the curriculum.

> I am dying with the help of too many physicians.
> —Alexander the Great, on his death-bed

We point out these changes and suggest that readers who need more in-depth knowledge of the physician education process do an aggressive web search. We strongly feel that a firm understanding of these processes will give additional insight in dealing with physicians.

THE TYPICAL CONTRAST BETWEEN PHYSICIANS AND ADMINISTRATORS

Kenneth Cohn (2008) wrote, "For physicians trained in the scientific method, problem solving is deductive and linear, leading to one best diagnosis and treatment. In general, physicians lose patience with an administrative approach that seeks multiple correct answers (options)."

> The dedicated doctor knows that he must be both scientist and humanitarian; his most agonizing decisions lie in the field of human relations.
> —David B. Allman, inaugural presidential address to the American Medical Association, June 1957

Providing management and leadership education is a challenge, given the differences between physicians and administrators. Most readers will recall seeing charts similar to the one in Exhibit 1.1, showing the contrast between physicians and administrators.

While great differences exist between physician and administrators, the two opposites must find ways to work together. This can be done through a better understanding of each other—which should be a foundation block of any development program—and by ensuring an adequate conflict management mechanism is in place organizationally (one of the topics of Chapter 8).

Exhibit 1.1: Characteristics of Physicians Versus Administrators

Physicians	Administrators
Science-oriented	Business-oriented
One-on-one interactions	Group interactions
Value autonomy	Value collaboration
Focus on patients	Focus on organization
Identify with profession	Identify with organization
Independent	Collaborative
Solo thinkers	Group thinkers

WHAT PHYSICIANS DO

Have you ever actually read the Hippocratic Oath? Here's the original—and not at all politically correct—Greek version translated into English:

> I swear by Apollo, the healer, Asclepius, Hygieia, and Panacea, and I take to witness all the gods, all the goddesses, to keep according to my ability and my judgment the following Oath and agreement:
>
> To consider dear to me, as my parents, him who taught me this art; to live in common with him and, if necessary, to share my goods with him; to look upon his children as my own brothers, to teach them this art; and that by my teaching, I will impart a knowledge of this art to my own sons, and to my teacher's sons and to disciples bound by an indenture and oath according to the medical laws, and no others.
>
> I will prescribe regimens for the good of my patients according to my ability and my judgment and never do harm to anyone.
>
> I will give no deadly medicine to any one if asked, nor suggest any such counsel; and similarly I will not give a woman a pessary to cause an abortion.
>
> But I will preserve the purity of my life and my arts.
>
> I will not cut for stone, even for patients in whom the disease is manifest; I will leave this operation to be performed by practitioners, specialists in this art.
>
> In every house where I come I will enter only for the good of my patients, keeping myself far from all intentional ill-doing and all seduction and especially from the pleasures of love with women or with men, be they free or slaves.

All that may come to my knowledge in the exercise of my profession or in daily commerce with men, which ought not to be spread abroad, I will keep secret and will never reveal.

If I keep this oath faithfully, may I enjoy my life and practice my art, respected by all humanity and in all times; but if I swerve from it or violate it, may the reverse be my life.

And here's the modern version, written in 1964 by Louis Lasagna, MD, one-time academic dean of the School of Medicine at Tufts University:

I swear to fulfill, to the best of my ability and judgment, this covenant:

I will respect the hard-won scientific gains of those physicians in whose steps I walk, and gladly share such knowledge as is mine with those who are to follow.

I will apply, for the benefit of the sick, all measures [that] are required, avoiding those twin traps of overtreatment and therapeutic nihilism.

I will remember that there is art to medicine as well as science, and that warmth, sympathy and understanding may outweigh the surgeon's knife or the chemist's drug.

I will not be ashamed to say "I know not," nor will I fail to call in my colleagues when the skills of another are needed for a patient's recovery.

I will respect the privacy of my patients, for their problems are not disclosed to me that the world may know. Most especially must I tread with care in matters of life and death. If it is given to me to save a life, all thanks. But it may also be within my power to take a life; this awesome responsibility must be faced with great humbleness and awareness of my own frailty. Above all, I must not play at God.

I will remember that I do not treat a fever chart, a cancerous growth, but a sick human being, whose illness may affect the person's family and economic stability. My responsibility includes these related problems, if I am to care adequately for the sick.

I will prevent disease whenever I can, for prevention is preferable to cure.

I will remember that I remain a member of society with special obligations to all my fellow human beings, those sound of mind and body as well as the infirm.

If I do not violate this oath, may I enjoy life and art, be respected while I live and remembered with affection thereafter. May I always act so as to preserve the finest traditions of my calling and may I long experience the joy of healing those who seek my help.

To what extent is this oath as relevant to new physicians today? Our challenge to our readers is to take this question on as an assigned homework project.

But what do physicians do? Consider the following discussions.

WHAT PHYSICIANS ARE LIKE

A lot has been said—maybe by you or a colleague—about how physicians relate to hospital administration. For example, "Doctors are soloists—but this too is changing." Or, "New physicians entering practice are different."

"Physicians have been trained and socialized to be fiercely independent. Practicing the art of medicine is a solo endeavor" (Wachter 2004). And yet, when considering Wachter's comment, successful physicians, even those few still in solo practice, have to get along with others, both in the community and in business situations.

Consider the following comment from John Morrissey (2010) regarding the impact of the new reform legislation: "The Patient Protection and Affordable Care Act, along with other economic forces and regulatory wrinkles, [is] driving physicians and hospital administrations into each other's arms, often for strategic reasons, but also for survival in the face of declining reimbursement. These forces will alter the ways hospitals and their physicians work with one another."

And meeting both sides' needs is possible (Lindberg and Paller 2008):

Physicians don't want to be treated solely as customers, nor do they wish to be considered team members like the rest of the hospital staff. Physicians need to be engaged in the planning process that supports and provides opportunities for their practices. Key drivers of physician relationships with hospital administrators include: planning for the future, ability to change, responsiveness to concerns and confidence, and trust. These drivers are what build and sustain a relationship that motivates physicians to refer patients to the facility, to comply with hospital guidelines and to share in the vision of the organization.

But readers should ask themselves, "To what extent am I viewing the physician world from the eyes of physicians who are in their late 40s and older?" These physicians grew up during the era of the soloist. Yet new residents scratch their heads at this notion and often state, "I was trained to be part of a team." Even traditional baccalaureate education for nonphysicians (business and social science majors, for example) includes many group and team assignments.

New physicians entering the workforce are focusing on different issues than their predecessors did. We no longer live in the world of Marcus Welby, and only one in four physicians plans to go into primary care. And those who move into internal medicine residencies usually end up specializing. Carrying large student loan debt has significantly changed the perspective of many new physicians. The newer generation also expects a balance of personal and work life. And finally, the personal economics of the earnings potential for various physician specialties continues to drive choices. Paul Keckley (2012b) reported that the "income disparity between primary care and specialty medicine continues to widen (per Medical Group Management Association, 2010 median compensation for primary care was $202,392 versus specialists at $356,885)."

It is the physician's pen that causes all motion in healthcare.
—*Quote from many healthcare administrators*

If you acknowledge some stern realities and some significant changes, you can see the importance of understanding the preparation of physicians in making a hospital–physician relationship (or a clinical integration organization) work.

SOME BRIEF THOUGHTS

Physicians have been pursued by hospitals and health systems to become close, and the twenty-first century opened with some experts reporting that practically two-thirds of all physicians had some type of arrangement with a hospital or health system (Zasa 2011). These arrangements range from income guarantees for recruitment to partnering on medical office buildings to joint ventures to comanagement models to outright employment by the hospital. The true solo physician is almost completely extinct. During the 1990s—when the industry predicted that reimbursement would lead to a capitated model requiring significant physician involvement in directing care—many organizations talked of creating "alignment" between physicians and hospitals or health systems. We think there has been much effort toward that but there are "miles to go before we sleep."

Many physicians continue to have connections to hospitals and health systems through medical staff committees, task forces, invitations to participate in strategic planning, and interaction with the physician relations staff. Even those physicians who practice exclusively outside of the acute care entities still interact with hospital-based specialists and often hospitalists.

A few organizations have become legendary in their synergy and connectedness with physicians. Many of these are clearly physician driven (e.g., Mayo Clinic, Cleveland Clinic), while others have begun innovative approaches to partnership (Advocate, Lehigh Valley Health Network, Heartland Health), and still others have strong alignment, cooperation, and connectedness because of specific interpersonal relationships among leaders from both sides. It is widely accepted in the field that organizations that have CEOs, COOs, and other senior executives who are open and inclusive with all physicians will have the strongest alignment. When this exists, all parties seem to sense the greater good, and the organization usually has higher quality and stronger operational and financial performance.

Finally, many partnerships spring from the relationships between physicians and the direct caregivers of a hospital or health system—the nurses, pharmacists, therapists, techs, and so forth. Team care and interdependence build strong relationships and ultimately benefit the greater partnership. This is increasingly having more impact on how physician management and leadership operate within the framework of the larger organization.

Later chapters will address the issue of collaboration more fully. Suffice it to say in this early chapter that collaboration is one key to enhanced physician leadership development.

Physician to Physician

Doctors are not a homogeneous group. In looking at how to achieve strategic management objectives, you have to be aware of the expectations for the different physician populations that are critical to the enterprise or organizational success as a whole. There is too often a tendency to say, "This guy is a doctor, so he will be overfocused on clinical and be totally impractical." But at the end of the day, that may be far from it. Those kinds of stereotypical characterizations will work against you in building effective leadership.
—Jacque Sokolov, MD

THE NEW BREED OF PHYSICIANS

Ask any physician recruiter today and you will hear details of a different group of physicians entering the workforce. As members of generations X/Y, the millennials, or whatever label is applied, these younger physicians are poles apart from their predecessors. The group's gender mix is more balanced—a little more than 50 percent of medical school graduates today are women. Younger physicians seek much more control over their work hours and personal lives; the issues of taking call and working weekends have become serious challenges for those staffing for patient care. With the advent of these needs, physicians have a greater interest in part-time schedules, job sharing, and different work patterns.

And one huge change stands out: Younger physicians want to be employed. These are not the doctors of the prior generation, who went into the private practice of medicine and essentially became small business owners. Many younger physicians come out of residencies with large student loans to repay and do not have the financial ability to buy into an existing practice. From 2000 to 2010, hospitals' physician employment jumped 32 percent to roughly 212,000 physicians (Bush 2012). What's more, the number of hospitals employing hospitalists rose from 29.6 percent in 2003 to 59.8 percent in 2010. That means hospitals now employ almost 20 percent of all physicians (Bush 2012).

Finally, physicians are working in larger and larger groups and settings and becoming more "institutionalized." "Physicians increasingly are practicing in mid-sized, single-specialty groups of six to 50 physicians" (Liebhaber and Grossman 2007).

Primary care has become less attractive and is less connected to the inpatient hospital enterprise. The rise of hospitalists has also changed the face of medicine significantly. From 2007 to 2010, the proportion of hospitals employing intensivists grew from 20.7 percent to 29.7 percent (Bush 2012).

CONCLUSION

No two physicians are exactly alike; that is just as true of them as it is of nonphysician healthcare administrators. Still, physicians do share many traits: their education is long, arduous, and focused on getting something done with a minimum of interference or outside input; they expect to control their professional destiny; and they recognize that they play a part in an increasingly complex healthcare system. Those key similarities are what healthcare administrators must be familiar with to maximize the value that physicians bring to the clinical integration table.

This chapter opens our discourse on physician leadership. Our purpose is to ask readers to take some time to ponder physicians and their nature. Physicians vary greatly in terms of practice, interests, and areas of focus. But to work best with them requires some fundamental understanding. Moreover, to presume to educate them in leadership demands an even greater understanding of their distinctiveness and hallmarks. Those charged with enhancing physician leadership must have a core understanding of physicians and the changes occurring in the physician population.

Thoughts for Consideration

Have you ever had a discussion with a physician about her educational background and professional history?

Do your institution's policies acknowledge the special place that physicians have in the healthcare community?

What do the specifics in the Hippocratic Oath tell you about physicians' perspective on hospital–physician relationships?

To what extent do the new and younger physicians entering the healthcare field believe in the oath?

Do you agree with the comments in "What Physicians Are Like"? Why or why not?

Is your institution prepared for the physicians of tomorrow and their evolving work–life demands?

How well do you know and understand physicians?

SUGGESTED READING

Cohn, K. H., S. L. Gill, and R. W. Schwartz. 2005. "Gaining Hospital Administrators' Attention: Ways to Improve Physician–Hospital Management Dialogue." *Surgery* 137 (2): 132–40.

Stevens, R. E., L. W. Lawrence, and D. Loudon. 1991. "The Public's Image of Doctors, Dentists and Pharmacists." *Health Marketing Quarterly* 9 (1–2): 97–105.

Note: Readers unfamiliar with the medical school and residency processes are encouraged to visit the website of the Association of American Medical Colleges (AAMC), www.aamc.org.

CHAPTER 2

Physician Engagement and Leadership: What Does It Mean?

At lunch during a national meeting of healthcare executives, five health system CEOs, two of whom were physicians, were in the midst of a spirited discussion about physician leadership.

CEO A: "I agree that physicians need to be more involved in leadership, but their real job is patient care and quality. To suggest that all healthcare organizations should have physicians running operations or in CEO positions is not logical."

CEO B: "I agree and, moreover, there are not enough physicians trained in finance and business to step up to the plate. I can understand having a chief medical officer, but the idea of physician COOs and CEOs just because the Cleveland Clinic and Mayo have them is not relevant to most systems."

CEO C: "I don't agree. Quite frankly, no one knows how the component parts of the healthcare system fit together better than a physician. I have had great success putting physicians in operations positions."

CEO D: "I have had similar experiences. I do feel that in the near future the real challenges we now face in healthcare are so complex that they will require a physician mind-set and many more physicians in direct line positions."

(continued)

> **CEO A:** "I'm not saying that physicians should not be involved—they should be—but not necessarily at the CEO or COO level. I think every strong healthcare organization needs a CMO. And I think that physicians should probably handle quality issues. But they just are not trained to be executives."
>
> **CEO E:** "Physicians should serve in leadership roles where they have the training and background, such as clinical areas and quality. In my opinion, they should steer clear of finance, marketing, and strategy."
>
> **CEO C:** "Other than some problems with semantics, I think we are all on the same page here. I think one of the key differences is that we who are physicians see a close link between clinical quality and business outcomes, such as financial performance and organizational effectiveness. I think we see these going hand in hand and not separate from one another. While it is certainly not logical to think that physicians are going to assume all leadership roles in healthcare organizations, I think we would all agree that their number is going to rapidly increase."

This opening vignette is intended to lead you on a mental journey down a road that ends with finding an answer to a key question: What does it mean to have physicians effectively involved and engaged in the leadership of the enterprise?

Some might phrase the question like this: "What does it mean to be physician led?" Others might suggest this: "How might we become more physician-centric?" No matter the nomenclature, addressing this question is critical before venturing too far into the nature of physician leadership.

We surveyed a number of healthcare leaders—both physicians and nonphysicians—asking this question, and the answers varied widely. The variation was rooted in a number of factors, including the following:

The type of organization. The answers will vary from organizations that are made up entirely of employed physicians to those that still have a large number of independent physicians. Physician leadership is different in an academic medical center than it is in a smaller rural hospital. In many small rural organizations, the only physicians in the region are those who are fully engaged in full-time clinical practice, and their leadership activities are quite part-time; an academic medical center will often have a physician CEO and full-time physician chairs who drive much of the activity of the entire organization. Both types of organizations could be viewed as physician led.

The type of issue confronted. The role of physician leadership will also differ according to the types of issues that the organization faces—for example, is the organization losing money and facing serious financial challenges, or is it facing clinical quality problems?

The emphasis on clinical integration. If one of the key strategies of the organization is clinical integration, then physician leadership is critical.

The history of the organization and its medical staff. If the organization has long had a well-developed and highly involved medical staff, it likely has a larger number of physician leaders.

The attitude of the organization's board and senior leadership toward physician involvement. Organizations that have long put a premium on actively involving physicians in setting strategy and making decisions are far down the road toward having strong physician leadership. Yet some organizations still have a view of physicians as being merely producers of the product, so they are given little input into the management and strategy decisions that drive the organization.

These and many other factors represent many points on a continuum of physician-centric or physician-led organizations. Over time, we see successful organizations moving more toward some form of physician-led reality. Our desire is to provide suggestions and guidance for every type of organization, ultimately giving support for enhanced physician leadership no matter which kind.

By *physician led*, we do not mean that organizations must have a physician CEO, COO, or even full-time physician managers or leaders. We mean simply that in physician-led organizations, physicians are actively involved in policymaking and strategy setting in some form and play a continuous role in the dynamic changes that occur in those organizations.

IS BEING PHYSICIAN LED A GOOD THING?

The context of our discussion presumes that being physician led is a *good* thing. We will leave it to readers to decide for themselves because we recognize that differences of opinion will exist. The reader must know, though, that the authors both believe physician-led healthcare organizations will usually have better clinical and quality outcomes, will be run more cost-effectively, and will have higher patient satisfaction. This does not necessarily mean that a physician-led organization has to have a physician CEO or even have full-time physician executives. We recognize the factors listed previously and realize that many variables make organizations quite different and, as a result, make the nature and scope of physician leadership in each one different. But

> The model of accountable care organizations that gives employers the most confidence is one led by a physician group partnered with a health plan.
> —*Victoria Stagg Elliott, 2011*

our premise throughout this book is that organizations will operate at a higher level with strong and active physician leadership and involvement.

Physician to Physician

Even in traditionally hospital-centric organizations, physician leadership is critical to achieving clinically integrated enterprise objectives going forward. Optimizing an enterprise's clinically integrated organization (CIO) and/or hospital functions is one thing, but physician leadership and active multistakeholder physician participation will ultimately spell success or failure for the enterprise as a whole.

The key premise of this book is that healthcare has evolved to the point that it needs *far more active, involved, and prepared* physician leaders, regardless of the type of organization or the nature of its challenges.

—Jacque Sokolov, MD

A final note regarding our prognostication: We believe that healthcare enterprises will be far more effective in quality, financial, and community measures by having far more full-time physician leaders and by placing many of them in active line-management roles.

Over time, organizations that are now composed partially or entirely of independent physicians practicing within the organization will continue to move to a pluralistic model of more employed physicians coexisting with the independent medical staff.

In the future, organizational entities will most likely employ the majority of physicians in some manner and have a large number of full-time, paid administrative leaders providing both management and leadership functions.

Physician to Physician

The medical director/chief quality officer is often evolving into the president or managing physician of a hospital-sponsored medical group. The ability to manage both financial and quality metrics is at the heart of value-based reimbursement.

—Jacque Sokolov, MD

A LOOK AT PHYSICIAN-LED ORGANIZATIONS

Examples of physician-led facilities are not hard to find. Indeed, some of the healthcare system's brightest lights have long been known for their physician-centric approach to hospital administration, and some recent additions to the list are applying what those established entities have learned to their own institutions. We chose several that have physician CEOs, although elsewhere in the book we will discuss organizations with nonphysician CEOs and other types of physician leaders.

Regional West Medical Center

Regional West Medical Center (RWMC) is one example of a physician-led organization. In 2006, RWMC, a 149-bed hospital in Scottsbluff, Nebraska, was having significant difficulty. Its long history of serving as a regional referral center was being challenged, and physician recruitment was difficult; in fact, the projected number of physicians in place was nearly 30 doctors below the level called for in RWMC's medical staff development plan. Critical access hospitals were having difficulty providing gateway services to RWMC because of that lack of physician access and availability, and so significant service volumes were going to northern Colorado. Had those trends continued, RWMC's position as a referral center would have deteriorated and become a small community hospital with a greatly diminished ability to serve its 70-mile footprint around Scottsbluff.

Todd Sorensen, MD, RWMC's chief executive officer, created a team of internal and external stakeholders to map out a course that would provide a comprehensive approach to the hospital's challenges. Working closely with the board of directors, hospital leadership, and medical staff, the team concluded that RWMC had three priorities to accomplish if it was to survive as a regional referral center. First, it needed a hospital-sponsored medical group to attract and retain physicians who didn't want to join smaller existing practices. Second, RWMC needed to create a clinical and economic model that allowed it to support healthcare services in its extended service area and more actively engage with surrounding critical access hospitals. Finally, it needed to create a management services organization (MSO) to help both medical group–based and independent physicians address critical infrastructure and technology needs to meet the increasing demands of government and private payers for quality and reporting requirements. Over a 16-month period, RWMC's physician leadership prioritized options, designed solutions, and led a multidisciplinary team that achieved successful outcomes. Indeed, the hospital-sponsored medical group grew from 0 to more than 60 physicians, and physician infrastructure development and supporting technology have grown enough that the Scottsbluff medical community is working with a major carrier to codevelop a regional ACO/medical home model.

Lehigh Valley Health Network

The Lehigh Valley Health Network (LVHN), based in Allentown, Pennsylvania, is another good example of a physician-led organization. Under CEO Ronald W. Swinfard, MD, the two-hospital system operates community health centers; an employed physician network of about 1,100; pharmacy, imaging, and home health services; a lab; and a health plan. The system even runs its own Institute for Physician Leadership (IPL), which is "designed to increase leadership, management, and professional capabilities through individual physician development" (LVHN 2008). As the LVHN website notes, "Today, the role of the physician increasingly demands more highly developed leadership and management skills. Physicians may find themselves exploring roles beyond that of an active clinician at Lehigh Valley Health Network—roles such as clinical medical program director, project leader, partner in a newly formed private practice, member of a research project team, committee chair of a governing group, director of a residency program, or board member of a not-for-profit community entity."

Under the program, department chairs and other senior leaders nominate physicians as IPL fellows (LVHN 2008). Physicians who accept the nomination commit to a two-year program of leadership development activities, including leadership cafés, forums, book clubs, and mentoring. Under the mentoring program, senior network physicians and administrators are paired with IPL fellows through a matching process. The institute is supported through a philanthropic grant, and there is no cost to the participating physician or to his or her practice aside from the commitment and management of time. Physicians also receive CME credits as fellows. The learning objectives of the institute are "to clarify informal and formal physician leadership roles, to understand the changing and increasingly competitive healthcare environment and the physician leader as a facilitative change agent in that environment, to broadly define how the physician leader can serve as a model for service and leadership excellence, and to develop a deeper understanding of leadership concepts, vocabulary, and organizational culture and function" (LVHN 2008).

East Jefferson General Hospital

Down near the Crescent City, in Metairie, Louisiana, East Jefferson General Hospital (EJGH) is embracing clinical integration, often a key goal of enhanced physician-led hospital administration. In an effort spearheaded by CEO and president Mark J. Peters, MD, CPE, EJGH has entered an ongoing collaborative relationship with the Gulf South Quality Network LLC (GSQN), a physician-managed, physician-operated, clinically integrated physician network that includes members from multiple medical, surgical, and primary care specialties. The GSQN's physician membership consists of "a select group of EJGH medical staff members who are either in independent practice or are employed by EJGH. All GSQN physician members have committed themselves to actively participating in ongoing efforts to maximize the value of healthcare services provided to their patients" (GSQN 2011). Clinical integration "is gaining momentum throughout the country as an effective way to provide care." Adds Peters: "East Jefferson knows that the future of healthcare requires the highest level of care coordination by all members of the medical community. We are proud that [more than] 200 physicians have already joined the GSQN, and we expect that number to continually grow. Through a sharing of resources, ideas and information, the newly established Gulf South Quality Network will allow East Jefferson General Hospital to deliver an even higher quality of care to our patients and our community" (GSQN 2011).

Cleveland Clinic

And then there are the big dogs. The Cleveland Clinic, the famous multispecialty academic medical center, was established as one of the first group practices—way back in 1921—by four physicians. Its current CEO is Toby Cosgrove, MD. Cleveland Clinic's roughly 2,500 staff physicians and residents now represent 120 medical specialties and subspecialties. It is the second-largest group practice in the world today, after the Mayo Clinic. Chief operating officer Marc Harrison, MD, explains, "A group model led by strong physician leaders can be very successful. When physicians are asked to do something, it resonates more when it comes from a doctor" (Page 2010). He concedes that "there are plenty of physician leaders who have done a terrible job running healthcare organizations." But he points out, "It does help to have management training, [and it is] important that the chief medical officer work closely with the CFO." Clinical integration also helps. "In the traditional healthcare organization," he explains, "heart surgeons and cardiologists, for example, are in different departments, work for different people, and have different business plans and separate profit and loss statements. And yet they have similar kinds of patients and they may even directly compete for some procedures, such as percutaneous heart valves. Combining these functions into one heart institute is easier to manage and easier for patients to understand" (Page 2010).

Mayo Clinic

The Rochester, Minnesota–based Mayo Clinic, the biggest group practice dog of them all, is a private group practice governed by physician-led committees. Mayo's president and CEO is neurologist John H. Noseworthy, MD. "While most other healthcare centers turn the management of their practices over to professional administrators, we stand by the philosophy that physician leadership keeps us grounded in the reason we are here—to provide the best care to every patient every day. Mayo Clinic physicians undertake rotating committee assignments where they partner with administrators to develop strategies and resolve problems because they understand the practice best. The strengths of this physician–administrator partnership have served Mayo Clinic well for the past century. Physician leadership ensures the preservation of our unique culture" (Mayo Clinic 2002). Indeed, one study's researchers determined that "physician leaders play vital roles in representing the interests of their physician colleagues and in balancing the needs of various stakeholders. Typical leader accountabilities and expectations include providing strategic direction and vision, evaluating program development, using resources to ensure alignment with organizational direction, ensuring the highest quality of care, enhancing professional competence and skill, developing and enforcing policies and procedures, and enhancing teamwork. Key to fulfillment of organizational expectations is the recruitment, career development, and retention of outstanding physicians" (Menaker and Bahn 2008).

Specifically, the researchers found, Mayo physician leaders "enhance their relationships with physicians by spending time teaching and coaching; treating physicians as individuals rather than just as members of the group; considering each individual as having different needs, abilities, and aspirations from others; and helping others to develop their strengths." And, the study report notes, "Physician leaders have an important role in shaping the healthcare system. They assume responsibilities that influence the design and success of the processes used to provide patient care [and they play] important roles in physician recruitment and career development. Physicians look to leaders for guidance in understanding the patient–physician relationship, one of life's most important partnerships. At Mayo Clinic, the responsibility of leaders to attract, develop, and retain the best faculty is considered a foundation of the organization's overall success in achieving its vision" (Menaker and Bahn 2008).

> **Physician to Physician**
>
> Physician leadership at the CEO level, while helpful, is not a guarantee of success unless the physician CEO possesses all the requisite governance, management, and operational capabilities consistent with those of her non-MD CEO colleagues.
> —Jacque Sokolov, MD

HOW WILL PHYSICIAN LEADERSHIP BE DEVELOPED?

We suggest that the reader consider our model of physician leadership and involvement. The ultimate goal is for an organization to improve patient quality and organizational effectiveness by promoting physician leadership.

Physician leaders will be developed through healthcare organizations' continuous progress in involving them. The model (see "Physician Leadership Development Model") shows specific factors that healthcare organizations should include as a part of their physician leadership and development programs.

Healthcare organizations should increase physician participation in governance, management, and strategic planning. They also should enhance physician and medical staff communications, optimize organizational structure, build better organization models for the identification and management of physician conflict, and develop physician relations programs.

Healthcare organizations must institute formal methods of identifying physician leaders and provide them with sound business, strategic, and administrative education. Managing quality and clinical integration are also key issues that organizations need to address to benefit from the increased role of physician leaders in driving quality outcomes. This practical approach is simple but is nonetheless an excellent audit guide for readers.

Physician Leadership Development Model

1. Identify physician leaders
2. Involve physicians in governance
3. Involve physicians in management
4. Involve physicians in strategic planning
5. Optimize organizational structure
6. Enhance physician communications
7. Manage physician conflict
8. Coordinate physician relations
9. Educate physician leaders
10. Manage quality and clinical integration

CONCLUSION

The future healthcare enterprise is one in which physicians will be actively involved in setting strategic direction and managing day-to-day operations. Ultimately, all the incentives will be aligned because the physician enterprise and the business enterprise that manages health, wellness, and sickness will be one and the same. The journey toward this future will require an increased emphasis on getting more physicians involved in steering the ship, helping to correct the course, and working with all areas of the endeavor.

Thoughts for Consideration

Which argument in the opening vignette sounds most like you?

To what extent is your organization physician led?

Which of the issues on pages 18–19 drive your organization's view of physician leadership?

Are you able to identify where on the physician-led continuum your organization is?

To what extent has your organization addressed the topic areas covered in the physician leadership and development model?

SUGGESTED READING

Correa, F. 2011. "Study: Top-Notch Hospitals Often Have Docs at Top." *Hospitalist News.* Posted July 22. www.ehospitalistnews.com/index.php?id=2050&type=98&tx_ttnews[tt_news]=61144&cHash=da03e20e36.

Page, L. 2010. "10 Tips to Creating a Physician-Led Integrated Care System with Advocate Health's Mark Shields." *Becker's Hospital Review.* Published September 14. www.beckershospitalreview.com/hospital-physician-relationships/10-tips-to-creating-a-physician-led-integrated-care-system-with-advocate-healths-mark-shields.html.

Riordan, M. 2011. "Physician Led." *To Transform Health Care.* Published August 14. http://totransformhealthcare.com/2011/08/physician-led/.

Part II

PHYSICIAN LEADERSHIP—
FIRST STEPS

CHAPTER 3

What We Have Learned

Learn all you can from the mistakes of others.
You won't have time to make them all yourself.
    —*Alfred Sheinwold*

> Highly effective organizations are learning organizations. Learning requires reflection on the past and study of both successes and failures. Effective physician leadership will improve patient safety and quality, financial performance, and community service. This chapter is unique because it represents the voices of many who have shared with us their successes and failures. It is intended to be a "sit back and listen" discourse providing insight and reflection from those who are active in the physician leadership arena.

We open with general observations about what we have learned.

The great divide must be bridged. A gulf still exists between physicians and administration in many organizations. Some of this is caused by conflicting priorities and goals, while some of it is caused by poor communications. But it remains.

Structures have hurt. Organizational structures—especially those that involve physician–hospital partnerships—are complex, often overly legalistic, and have not provided good exchange between physicians and leadership. While we recognize that structures such as joint ventures or comanagement models have served in some cases to bring physicians and healthcare organizations to the table, the overarching theme of these models is economic. And if money is the only thing to talk about, stress is guaranteed when the size of the money pie decreases.

Leading physicians is challenging. Physicians, as a class of people, are exceptionally bright, were often at the top of their classes, and have been trained in a highly competitive environment. These factors make leading physicians a challenge.

But physicians can be led. And engaged. And in sync with the mission and vision of the organization. Many organizations have succeeded in engaging their physicians and building them into a cohesive and supportive team.

Physicians' manner of learning is different. Physicians like to learn the way they are trained—through hands-on activities. "Learn and do" is the mantra for physician education. Therefore, physician leadership development cannot be as classroom-oriented as it is for other individuals.

Physicians do not typically work in teams. The medical school and residency years and the typical clinical practice have physicians functioning as independent professionals. Even physicians who work in group practices do most of their clinical work on their own. In their work, they typically are decisive and at times dictatorial. Performing in teams can be difficult. One observer suggested that getting a group of physicians together was akin to having all the quarterbacks in a league come together to establish a team—it is just not a likely scenario.

Communication continues to be a great challenge. Our observations and experiences suggest that communication challenges are not caused by a *lack* of communications. Practically all organizations have ample communications vehicles and use many different methods to communicate with physicians. However, because physicians vary so greatly in their motives, needs, and issues, the need to customize communications becomes an even greater imperative. Moreover, the issues often involve confused messages, mixed messages, and perceptions that favorites exist within the physicians collective.

Physician leadership development programs have not often succeeded. The highly effective programs are few in number. We believe that much of the lack of success is tied to the heavy emphasis on classroom training.

Too much leadership is done by those at the end of their careers. The usual physician leaders are veteran individuals with lots of career experiences, and they often do not represent the full spectrum of physicians (either by age or by specialty).

> The past is behind, learn from it.
>
> The future is ahead, prepare for it.
>
> The present is here, live it.
> —Thomas S. Monson

Phrases like "herding cats" do not serve the effort positively. We consciously avoid using this often-heard phrase because we do not accept or believe it. Phrases such as this create a negative environment, fail to be constructive, and cause a distorted representation of reality.

Physician apathy may be one of the greatest arguments for enhanced physician leadership. Many individuals have talked to us of the current state of physician apathy: "Physicians just are not like they used to be—we always had leaders who would step up to the plate and lead the medical staff." This habit of lamenting the current times and longing for the good old days is counterproductive.

SURVEY OF PHYSICIANS

In May 2012, we conducted a brief survey to determine what we have learned about physician leadership. The results are provided below and represent the thoughts of several physician chief medical officers, vice presidents of medical affairs, and CEOs.

Survey Results Detail

From a professional (leadership) development standpoint, describe in a few words what you as a physician leader have learned from your biggest success—and how that has changed the way you analyze issues at your institution.

1. Identifying key physician "players" early in the process and deciding how they receive information and their required level of involvement is essential. In doing this, I have learned that success comes faster and engagement is more inclusive.
    ◆ If you decide on certain consequences for certain actions, you need to enforce them.
    ◆ Rather than dwell on trying to anticipate what the reaction to strategic initiatives is going to be from the physicians, I create a logical explanation as to why what we are trying to accomplish is important, I directly ask for support, and I don't avoid debating the merits, acknowledging that no plan is perfect, but we cannot stay in the status quo.
    ◆ Welcome criticism and incorporate constructive criticism into the final product. Communicate draft proposals broadly to physician leaders in a way that solicits feedback early.
    ◆ Be quick to listen, slow to speak, and even slower to get angry.
    ◆ Engaging physicians at the medical staff leadership or performance improvement level, not only as required by The Joint Commission (credentialing and periodic performance review) but in every aspect of hospital operations that impacts physicians, is necessary for organizational excellence. Most physicians do not leave medical school or postgraduate training with the skills for managing engagement, so additional train-

ing is necessary. Some call it resocialization. This can be extrapolated to the more than 95 percent of leaders at any healthcare organization [who] went into healthcare for reasons other than management. They frequently do not have the tools to manage. An organizational commitment to giving them these tools and holding them accountable for their use is also necessary for success. We do both at [our organization].

- What's in it for me is still very important!
- In my 11 years here, building trust so that physician leaders feel they have support for the "crucial conversations" is imperative. The biggest successes result from being able to make big decisions and successfully implement them. To do so, just about everyone has to be pulling in the same direction.
- Culture eats strategy.
- Alignment of incentives (financial, political, and personal) up and down the chain, and solid communications and buy-in/ownership of all players are key to any success.
- Share the wealth, include everybody up front, and deflect praise to others.
- Risk taking, leading innovation, different perspective[s] allow for competitive differentiation.

2. From a professional (leadership) development standpoint, describe in a few words what you—as a physician leader—have learned from your biggest failure and how you think or manage things differently as a result.
   - Unless you have buy-in, you will fail.
   - Don't get out too far in front. Make sure that you give people time to assimilate what you are trying to accomplish and get on board.
   - Often too much detail and information are not needed. Physicians tend to want to be heard, speak in summation from the onset, and become disengaged if the detail does not have value in their decision process.
   - You can't be afraid to have the difficult conversation with a colleague.
   - Trying to get everyone on the same page is a big waste of time and will only stall or kill a project.
   - Violating my own "rules." Bringing open-ended questions to physician committees populated by 15 different specialties will usually get the wrong answer eight to seven. Medical meetings should be run like a company board, with the appropriate stakeholders on board before

the meeting, so that issues can be addressed efficiently without everyone in the room discoursing on the first thought after hearing the issue. The couple of times I have violated this rule because I perceived a more pressing time pressure have reinforced its importance.

- Be inclusive when planning for change.
- There is no amount of ink and legal advice that can compensate for shared goals and incentives, no matter what the organizational structure.
- With each decision there are intended and unintended consequences. I always consider the unintended consequences.
- Before embarking on any effort to make real changes, make sure you have not only buy-in, but solid commitment from the "top critical decision makers" or key stakeholders that if indeed you can successfully put all the elements in place, they are willing to pull the trigger and not flip-flop or renege after much effort and convincing proof. Also make sure that the "stated" goals are also the "real" goals—not a surrogate.
- It's not about one thing; it is about the continuum, and never stop trying to improve.
- Not spending enough time developing relationships and instead being focused on getting the task done.

3. On a scale of 1 to 5, with 1 being "Disagree Strongly" and 5 being "Agree Strongly," how would you answer these questions?
   - [3a] Administrators trained as administrators will always do a better job of running a healthcare organization than administrators trained as clinicians.

Strongly Disagree	Disagree	Neither Disagree nor Agree	Agree	Strongly Agree
1	2	3	4	5

   - [3b] Clinical integration at healthcare organizations is mission critical moving forward, and physicians must be part of the leadership that makes it happen.

Strongly Disagree	Disagree	Neither Disagree nor Agree	Agree	Strongly Agree
1	2	3	4	**5**

- [3c] It is important to find leaders with expertise in the specific tasks and functions we need to focus on, no matter what kind of background they have.

Strongly Disagree	Disagree	Neither Disagree nor Agree	Agree	Strongly Agree
1	2	**3**	4	5

General comments from the survey about physician leadership development:

- Content expertise is not nearly as important as cultural fit and credibility.
- Our yearly physician leadership training involves a real project in which physicians have skin in the game and includes management working alongside. All executive team members are alums of the physician leadership course.
- One of the biggest obstacles for physicians is adjusting one's event horizon from a 15- to 40-minute clinical encounter to a realistic organizational impact time line. This can be seen in physicians' needing to respond to an e-mail NOW instead of parking it and responding effectively a day later, or needing to come up with some solution at a meeting so the idea can be off their radar until the patient's next visit.
- Physicians have waited too long to retake an active role in leadership. It is critical for physicians to be trained in administrative process and blend sound business sense with patient-centered care for our patients. We can no longer think about "my patient(s)" but must focus on sustaining a healthcare system for all patients.
- Someone has to pay attention to this for physicians with significant leadership roles. No matter what level of natural leadership talent a physician may have, there is substantial benefit from training for a specific job. And great clinicians do not always make great leaders because many of the talents required are different. So it's worth spending some money training physicians.
- You need to start at the bottom—first going to committees, then department chair, then medical staff leadership; if it still interests you, then get educated and network for full-time work. It is an easier task to get full-time work at your own institution, assuming you were viewed as a good clinician, because that gives you credibility with the medical staff. This can be harder to establish from the outside.

- For a physician leader to be truly successful interacting outside the clinical walls, she must have knowledge of payer (government/employer) and health plan (benefit design, revenue stream, contracting, etc.) functions/limitations to successfully contract and have realistic expectations.
- This requires physicians to learn and practice a completely new set of skills. It is a process that takes years.

I am always ready to learn, although I do not always like being taught.
—*Winston Churchill, 1952*

OUR VIEW ON PHYSICIAN LEADERS AS A WHOLE

Truly successful physician leaders have prepared themselves—through a combination of additional study and education as well as management and leadership experiences—to manage and lead effectively. Many have gained advance management degrees (such as MBA, MHA, MPH, or JD) while others have had strong nonphysician leadership mentors. None of them feel that they are in their position solely because of their physician education and practice experiences.

Moreover, these strong physician leaders have honed key leadership competencies and practiced positive interpersonal relations with others. Although they have had little to no education in leadership and interpersonal skills development, they have picked it up somehow.

The work of clinicians differs from that of managers and leaders. Clinicians work directly with patients, they make decisions quickly (many spend just seven to ten minutes with a single patient), and they rely on independent judgment and skills to do their job. This work is not the job of a manager or leader and must be fully realized when developing a physician leadership program.

Thoughts for Consideration

Do you have a sense of how your physicians feel about leadership opportunities for themselves and other physicians?

To what extent is the physician leadership development program in your organization strategic (as opposed to tactical)?

Have you ever asked physicians the questions discussed in this chapter?

Our thanks to the members of The Healthcare Roundtable—the Physician CEO Roundtable and the Chief Medical Officer Roundtable—for their input on this chapter.

CHAPTER 4

Identification of Physician Leaders

Bruce Boling, vice president of medical affairs: We are constantly looking for potential physician leaders, typically younger members of our medical staff who show natural leadership characteristics. Once we identify someone, we have several conversations with her to gain a better sense of long-term personal and professional goals. Occasionally, I will take one with me to some committee meetings, and if there is some interest in leadership shown, I will then take a few of them with me to a national conference.

Jane Curtin, CEO: We use our Physician Leaders Academy to help identify future physician leaders. We have a six-month course, "Introduction to Management," that is offered to any physician interested in getting more involved in leadership roles. Our elected medical staff supported the academy by requiring that any physicians wanting to move into an elected office take the course.

Mary Rodriguez, CEO: Our board holds an annual discussion on physician leadership. We review those who have been in leadership positions and those who are about to move into them. We also discuss our leadership development programs and those in our up-and-comers group who will soon surface as new physician leaders.

Bob Younger, CEO: I hate to say it, but we really do not have a process to select our physician leaders. Our medical staff feels that selecting leaders is their job and we should stay out of it. In some respects, that used to be OK, but now that we employ a larger percentage of our medical staff, we need to insert ourselves more aggressively into the leader selection process.

Jeff Dubowski, chief medical officer: I am pleased to hear that all of you at least have some approach to identifying physician leaders, but my concern is that even with a formal process to do so, there simply are not enough candidates to fill the spots that we are going to need as we make our shift to clinical integration.

Identification of Physician Leaders

Contemporary organizations have formalized methods to identify physician leaders. They include a methodical procedure to prospect for potential leaders; a process for selecting physician leaders; a naming process, so those who are identified and respected as potential leaders know of their selection; and an awareness campaign, which indicates the importance of physician leadership within the organization. These organizations also use a well-developed leadership competency model to help identify potential leaders. Most organizations also have developed a method to help these prospective physician leaders understand the challenges and rewards of leadership and to have the chance to try their hand at involvement at the leadership level.

This chapter discusses the important process of identifying physicians who have the motivation and ability to move into leadership roles—a matter often overlooked by many organizations. Essentially, this process is the first step of the Physician Leadership Development Model introduced in Chapter 2. To give physicians a more active leadership role in the new paradigm of the healthcare world, healthcare organizations must make a concerted effort to recognize and single out physicians who will be recruited to leadership positions. Put simply:

How are physician leaders identified?

Healthcare industry administrators train to move into leadership positions. Increasing numbers of graduate programs in health administration as well as traditional MBA programs offer courses in leadership. Practically all graduates from these programs will indicate that one motivation for earning the degree is to "move into leadership positions." Yet, in their academic preparatory programs, physicians do not take such courses. Nor do physicians typically contemplate organizational leadership roles as they begin their careers. Physicians also often just fall into leadership positions. In some organizations, the joke is that physicians nominated for leadership positions were out of the room when the nominations occurred. Overall,

Exhibit 4.1: The Process of Identifying and Selecting Potential Physician Leaders

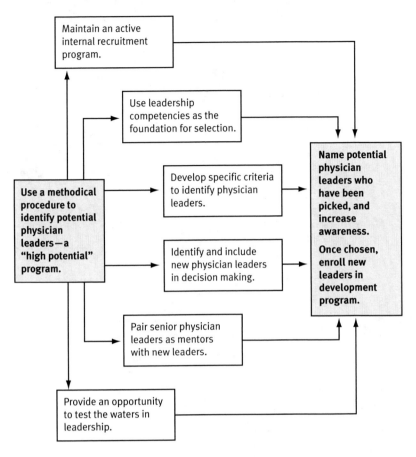

physicians' training and career paths do not automatically provide a way to naturally progress toward leadership roles. Because of these factors, establishing a process to identify physician leaders is critically important for organizations.

An excellent overview of a strategic approach to identifying physician leaders is provided in Exhibit 4.1. The model shows the critical importance of approaching the issue from a holistic viewpoint. Readers are encouraged to use the model and the material in this chapter to raise the bar in getting physician leadership to a more effective level in their organizations.

How might organizations go about this task? "Identifying Physician Leaders" shows the components of successful physician leadership identification.

Identifying Physician Leaders

To identify potential physician leaders, use a methodical procedure that

- identifies the competencies that are desirable for leadership and recognizes that these competencies form the foundation for any physician leadership development activities;
- develops specific criteria to identify potential physician leaders and uses them to recruit those potential leaders;
- commits to an ongoing, active internal program for recruiting physician leaders;
- names physician leaders who have been selected and increases awareness of physician leadership as a priority in the organization;
- allows both part-time and full-time involvement in management and leadership;
- includes both formal and informal physician leaders in programs, decision-making bodies, and policy discussions;
- provides specific information on what it means (in terms of time commitment, educational preparation, remuneration, growth opportunities, and areas for involvement) to be a physician leader in the organization;
- establishes a mentoring program that pairs senior physician leaders and other senior leaders with new physician leaders; and
- informs physicians that they have been chosen for leadership positions or identified as potential leaders.

Physician to Physician

This is not the time to select the chair or president for a physician leadership position because he did not show up for the meeting. Almost every doctor has been made a chair by not attending a meeting at some point. It is important that core competencies related to physician leadership should be the guiding principles for selection. And with the typical first-time physician leadership position, two key competencies are respect within the physician community and skill at relating interpersonally with other physicians to deal with the task at hand.
—*Jacque Sokolov, MD*

TRADITIONAL SELECTION OF LEADERS

How do healthcare organizations typically identify physician leaders? Consider the following:

1. **Self-nomination.** This is likely the most frequent way that physicians have historically surfaced in leadership, particularly in the voluntary medical staff model. At times—fortunately—this method provided effective leadership for the medical staff, but at other times it did not.
2. **Reward for loyalty.** Many organizations recognize physicians who are loyal by sponsoring them for leadership positions.
3. **"She looks like a leader."** As a reason for choosing leaders in areas outside the physician world, the illusion that leaders simply stand out among others continues to exist. While there may be some credence to this, placing an inordinate amount of weight on this factor can be dangerous.
4. **"Grievance docs."** Along the same lines as self-nomination, noted above, some physicians have certain issues, gripes, or complaints and insert themselves into leadership positions to address them.
5. **"My time has come."** This method is the classic appointment process—often for someone who was out of the room and not really seeking a leadership position—and it still exists in many voluntary medical staffs today.

Historically, however, the main criterion used to advance physicians into leadership positions has been their clinical accomplishments (much the same as in nursing and other clinical disciplines). "He is a great doctor; therefore, he will be a great medical staff president." This age-old assumption continues to harm many efforts to get the right people in leadership positions.

USING LEADERSHIP COMPETENCIES TO AID SELECTION

Clearly, these means of finding physician leaders are no longer acceptable. Given the uncertain environment in healthcare organizations today, leaders must be chosen in a more rational and methodical manner. Formal leader identification programs will supplant these ineffective methods of leadership selection. Instead of saying, "She looks like a leader" or "That physician seems like he could be a strong leader," enlightened organizations today are using more structured approaches to the identification and selection process. The most effective organizations use leadership competency models as a basis of their leadership programs. For a concise definition of competencies, see "What Are Competencies?" Competencies can be used to guide organizations as they identify those physicians who have leadership potential.

What Are Competencies?

Competencies are "a broad collection of knowledge, skills, abilities, and characteristics. They include values (such as ethics and integrity), cognitive skills (such as thinking and problem solving), interpersonal skills (such as communicating and listening), embracing diversity (such as tolerance and respect), and change management (such as strategic planning and risk taking)" (Dye and Garman 2006).

In their book *Exceptional Leadership: 16 Critical Competencies for Healthcare Leaders* (2006), Carson Dye and Andrew Garman present a clear model of leadership competencies. The model is easily used and provides an excellent framework for identifying potential physician leaders. More important, the model focuses on the specific competencies that set apart truly exceptional leaders from merely good ones. According to this model, exceptional leaders are strong in the following areas:

- Well-cultivated self-awareness
  - Living by personal conviction
  - Possessing emotional intelligence
- Compelling vision
  - Being visionary
  - Communicating vision
  - Earning loyalty and trust
- Real way with people
  - Listening like you mean it
  - Giving feedback
  - Mentoring others
  - Developing teams
  - Energizing staff
- Masterful execution
  - Generating informal power
  - Building consensus
  - Making decisions

- Driving results
- Stimulating creativity
- Cultivating adaptability

Deeper analysis of these competencies indicates that physician leaders need to be particularly strong in the following areas:

- **Building consensus.** Perhaps one of the more important skills that new and seasoned physician leaders use frequently is the ability to build consensus between different types of physicians as well as physicians and nonphysicians, uniting entire organizations around goals such as a focus on improved patient care or clinical outcomes.

- **Earning loyalty and trust.** Although an argument could be made that employed physicians are more willing to follow their leaders, the nature of physicians' work with patients (in which they generally assume sole responsibility) typically makes most physicians far more independent than other people. Therefore, physicians may be less willing to trust others or work in teams. Physician leaders must be able to apply the skills of building loyalty and trust in their interactions as leaders as well as their work as clinicians.

- **Living by personal conviction and possessing emotional intelligence.** Although these two competencies may seem obvious for leaders, they are paramount in discerning who will be strong physician leaders and who will likely not be able to make the transition to a leadership role.

- **Cultivating adaptability.** The ability to deal with all types of physicians, constantly changing priorities, and the significant complexities of healthcare organizations and the healthcare field requires flexibility and a contingent style of leadership (which posits that leadership behaviors are always contingent on three primary variables: the leader, the followers, and the situation).

As discussed in Chapter 1 on the nature of physicians, some characteristics of leadership do not lend themselves to quantitative description. Much of medicine is scientific. When it comes to making many leadership decisions, as one CEO pointed out, "Consensus is a political process, while science is an evidentiary process." In other words, leadership decisions are often subjective and provide multiple solutions, while medical decisions are more objective and typically have a single solution.

A more detailed look at the use of competencies as they relate to selection is presented in Chapter 12.

CRITERIA TO HELP IDENTIFY POTENTIAL PHYSICIAN LEADERS

This section provides insight into the types of criteria that can be used to identify those physicians who are not yet in leadership positions but possibly should be recruited or persuaded to consider physician leadership roles.

Although it may seem quite logical to do so, many organizations do not use any formal criteria to identify potential physician leaders. We are in essence suggesting that the following question be asked—and answered:

If I were going to select a group of physicians who had the best probability of assuming leadership positions and becoming effective leaders, what criteria would I use to select them?

We suggest using the following criteria:

- **Their clinical and service calling.** Potential physician leaders should be better-than-average clinicians, highly dedicated to the mission of caring for others, and interested in continual learning.
- **Their ethical and interpersonal calling.** Potential physician leaders should have high ethical principles, be individuals who stand up for what they believe, and serve as role models. They should not be driven by visions of personal glory, rank, status, or privilege, or by the ego satisfaction that comes with managing others. They also should understand that leadership is an ethical duty that requires service to the people being led.
- **Their leadership calling.** Potential physician leaders should be interested in broad strategic matters. They should be excited about the vision of healthcare and issues broader than their own practices, apply that vision to themselves, and look to add value to an organization. They should have the ability to get others to cooperate and do things together; essentially, they should be able to lead a group effectively.
- **Their traits.** The "potentials" should be persons of high integrity, authenticity, and fair-mindedness. They should be servant leaders who walk the talk, are focused on improvement, and are able to communicate effectively (clearly, precisely, succinctly, and in an engaging and compelling manner).
- **Match with leadership competencies.** Highly effective organizations also use their leadership competency models to evaluate entrance into leadership ranks. As discussed earlier in this chapter, a competency model can form the basis of selection.

RECRUITING HIGH-POTENTIAL PHYSICIAN LEADERS

"We need a lot of physician leaders, and one way we find these leaders is by taking a close look at the physicians who serve on our management committees for each specialty or geographic market."

—*Jon Kluge, vice president of clinical operations at Aurora Medical Group (Sloan and Fralicx 2011)*

Another way to ensure the right physicians are chosen for leadership positions is to develop a recruiting-style approach. First, organizations should identify individuals (typically current physician leaders, the CEO, and other seasoned executives) who can make themselves available to talk to physicians who might have interest in leadership roles. Contemporary organizational leadership concepts call these individuals "high potentials." Perhaps the best definition of a high potential is the one used by the Corporate Leadership Council (2005): "An employee who is assessed as having the ability, organizational commitment, and motivation to rise to and succeed in more senior positions in the organization." As authors, we cannot think of a better definition to use when considering those high-potential physicians who might be able to make a significant impact in an organizational leadership position.

As mentioned earlier in this chapter, some physicians will naturally present themselves for leadership positions. Yet these may not be the right people to assume those roles. Thus the organization must have some criteria established to minimize this dilemma. Some organizations require elected medical staff officers to take some type of leadership courses (the Physician in Management Seminar [PIMS] program with the American College of Physician Executives often is used) as a condition of assuming the elected role.

Simply articulating and putting forward the various motivations that different physicians have for moving into leadership positions is also important. "Right" reasons and "wrong" reasons for moving into leadership positions exist. Exhibit 4.2 provides some insight. Having these reasons on the table often helps when dealing with a headstrong or problematic doctor who wants a leadership role for the wrong reason.

LEADERS OR MANAGERS

Although the terms *management* and *leadership* are often used interchangeably, for the purposes of this discussion (and for many of the discussions within this book), noting the differences is important. The motivation for physicians to move

Exhibit 4.2: Right and Wrong Reasons Physicians Choose to Become Leaders

Right Reasons	Wrong Reasons
◆ To affect healthcare on a broader level ◆ To improve patient safety and quality ◆ To become part of the decision-making process ◆ To introduce and make change and to lead strategy ◆ To further personal growth ◆ To be inducted by the organization as a high-potential leader	◆ To "coast" into retirement ◆ To reduce work hours (eliminate call or weekend coverage) ◆ To exit a practice that has grown tiresome ◆ For physical reasons (such as being no longer able to take the physical strain) ◆ Personal agenda (the wrong one)

into different roles may be tied to either (a) an interest in "fixing" something in a department or area, which is a management issue, or (b) a broad-brush desire to make significant changes to an organization or a system, which is a leadership issue. Understanding the differences may be helpful in holding preliminary discussions with physicians who are considering management or leadership roles.

Note that within the context of this discussion, the authors believe that *both* management and leadership are important to the success of an organization; we do not subscribe to the popular theory that leadership is more important than management. Organizations need physicians who will take the day-to-day *management* positions in which decisions have direct impact on quality, cost, and service as well as physicians who think strategically and longer term to take on broader and more strategic *leadership* roles.

Note the differences in focus (see Exhibit 4.3). Many physicians move into what we will call administrative positions (which covers under its umbrella both management and leadership roles) by taking charge of some area or project. They become

Exhibit 4.3: Management and Leadership Positions for Physicians

Possible Management Positions for Physicians	Possible Leadership Positions for Physicians
◆ Physician chief of an intensive care unit ◆ Physician manager of a cardiac cath lab ◆ Supervisor of a hospitalist program	◆ Physician CEO ◆ Board positions ◆ System chief medical officer

section chiefs or run part of a lab or become part-time medical directors in charge of ongoing review of an area. Many physicians experience their first move out of clinical practice through this route, by managing their office practices or hospital departments or divisions. Yet other physicians find themselves in positions that deal with broad organizational issues that are strategic and longer term in nature. Often this involvement is through becoming members of their organizations' boards or being asked to participate in strategic planning retreats. The competencies required for these different kinds of leadership and management roles are also different. In the job that is more day-to-day management, the competencies involved are organizing, facilitating, and communicating, while in the more strategic positions, the competencies involved are strategic visioning, persuading, and change management. When recruiting physicians into leadership roles, making some distinctions in this sphere is important.

The importance of understanding the differences between physicians in management positions and physicians in leadership positions (and of course, those who do both) is provided in Chapter 5.

INCLUDING PHYSICIANS IN PROGRAMS, DECISION-MAKING BODIES, AND POLICY DISCUSSIONS

Another excellent way to expose potential physician leaders to leadership is to get them involved in organizational programs and seated on committees or other organizational structures that affect organizational management and leadership. Given the dramatic increase in development of clinically integrated organizations (CIOs), multiple governance, management, and operating physician leadership opportunities exist. At the governance level, physicians will be needed to serve on the board of directors. At the senior leadership level, physicians and nonphysicians will be needed to lead meaningful clinical integration. Last, at the operating level, multiple physician managers will be needed to focus on value-based care, value-based quality, and value-based financial performance.

An excellent first step for the physician exploring management and leadership is getting involved in medical staff committees. Participation in the medical staff's leadership and committee structure, including the medical executive committee and department or division chairs, provides an excellent insight into Joint Commission requirements that involve physician participation and expand the emerging physician leader's knowledge of hospital operations.

Special task forces or program development teams represent another avenue of involvement. The creation of centers of excellence, service line projects, and disease-specific care pathways all provide emerging physician leaders with the opportunity to combine clinical content expertise with emerging management integration required for successful execution of these programs. Examples in which physicians have led significant initiatives include women's health Centers of Excellence, neuroscience service line development, and complex congestive heart failure care pathways.

Quality and systems improvement efforts of Lean enterprise and Six Sigma provide excellent opportunities for involvement. Physicians are often called on to chair enterprisetwide board quality committees, medical staff quality committees, and institute-level quality committees. In addition, physicians are becoming increasingly knowledgeable about work process improvement, including Lean and Six Sigma programs that require the physician to understand quality issues and work process efficiencies.

Physician Mentoring Programs

Mentoring is best defined as a formal program whereby, typically, individuals who are more seasoned in leadership positions provide guidance to less-seasoned persons. While mentoring often involves counsel and coaching on specific management and leadership problems, it can also entail giving insight into the nature of a leadership position. Many physicians first considering leadership roles ask questions such as "What do I need to know to handle this role?" and "Should I get a master's degree to help me deal with these problems?"

For physicians who are uncertain about their desire to move out of clinical practice toward a more administrative role, mentors can provide many benefits, such as the following:

♦ A better understanding of the nature of leadership and the challenges faced
♦ Insight into the types of skills and competencies needed for success in leadership by coaching, counseling, listening, and modeling
♦ Knowledge about avenues into management and leadership roles and positions
♦ Awareness about how leaders influence change
♦ Insight into the time commitments involved in these positions

And for physicians who have just moved into their first management or leadership position, mentors can provide the following benefits:

- Guidance that ensures a smoother transition into the leadership position
- Career development advice (e.g., what courses to take or the benefits of various types of master's degree programs)
- A complement to formal study programs
- Different perspectives on management and leadership issues
- Insight and suggestions on management problems
- Broader networking into a leadership group

"When They Are Picked, Let Them Know!"

As simple as this may sound, it is important: Physicians who are identified as potential leaders need to be made aware of their selection. If the organization makes the first step in naming a potential physician leader, she needs to know this, and the organization should ensure that she knows the reasons for her selection. Conversely, if a physician takes initiative to express interest in a leadership position and is picked, the organization needs to communicate that decision as well.

Many organizations outside healthcare are known for their internal leadership selection programs. One of the better examples is Procter & Gamble (P&G). The Center for Management Research (2010) aptly describes the efforts of A. G. Lafley, former CEO of P&G, to develop a companywide leadership development process that encompasses areas such as selection, training, and individual assessment. This well-run corporation has a "build from within" policy as well as a "talent portfolio" that contains a list of upcoming leaders at the company. The key aspect of this program is that it is well known within P&G that these individuals have been identified for higher-level leadership positions. This step serves both as special recognition of these individuals and as a way to segment them to take on greater responsibility.

The Leadership Pipeline program at Wells Fargo (2012), the Knowledge Intensive University at DuPont (Cooper 2000), and the well-known General Electric Crotonville program (General Electric 2012) also place high emphasis on ensuring that newly identified up-and-coming leaders are recognized and acclaimed.

This process also provides a recognition feature. Acknowledgment is known to be a strong motivator. One Midwestern hospital provides special recognition on an annual basis to physicians who have handled special leadership positions. While most organizations provide some form of thank-you recognition to departing medical staff elected officers, this organization also gives recognition to physicians who have played any type of leadership role (e.g., committee chair, board committee membership, physician board member, IT conversion committees).

Generating publicity about physicians who are identified as potential and up-and-coming leaders also contributes to the development of a physician-led culture discussed in Chapter 2.

The bottom line is that highly effective organizations have well-structured leadership development programs, but also incorporate a step that identifies and recognizes potential leaders. Executing this step also ensures that others within the organization know the critical importance of physician leadership.

CONCLUSION

Building a physician leadership bench does not happen haphazardly. There must be a concerted effort to monitor the physician collective to assess and identify those from within who might be worthy physician leaders for the organization. This is job one in starting to build a high-performance physician leadership development program.

Thoughts for Consideration

Does your organization understand the multiple levels of need related to physician leadership participation—governance, management, and operations—especially the levels of need related to clinically integrated organizations?

To what extent does your organization actively try to identify potential leaders?

Are there individuals within your organization with whom a physician could visit to discuss potential interest in leadership?

Do you have a prepared response for them to give and a demonstrable leadership development program?

Are mentors provided to potential and new physician leaders?

Is there a formal, structured mentoring program in place?

Has your organization developed criteria for selection of potential physician leaders?

Do physicians know those criteria and the potential rewards of meeting them?

SUGGESTED READING

Avakian, L. 2011. "On the Hospital Agenda: Developing Physician Leaders." *Hospitals & Health Networks.* Published July 7. www.hhnmag.com/hhnmag/HHNDaily/HHNDailyDisplay.dhtml?id=1840006642.

Byham, W. C., A. B. Smith, and M. J. Paese. 2002. *Grow Your Own Leaders: How to Identify, Develop, and Retain Leadership Talent.* Upper Saddle River, NJ: FT Press.

Cantlupe. J. 2011. "Developing Empathetic Physician Leaders." *Health Leaders Media.* Published July 28. www.healthleadersmedia.com/page-1/PHY-269130/Developing-Empathetic-Physician-Leaders.

Dye, C. F. 2002. *Winning the Talent War: Ensuring Effective Leadership in Healthcare.* Chicago: Health Administration Press.

Dye, C. F., and A. N. Garman. 2006. *Exceptional Leadership: 16 Critical Competencies for Healthcare Executives.* Chicago: Health Administration Press.

Fritz, A. L., T. Sagin, and R. A. Sheff. 2003. *How to Recruit and Develop Physician Leaders: A Strategy for Medical Staff Leadership Development.* Danvers, MA: HCPro, Inc.

Linney, B. J. 2006. *A Career Guide for Physician Executives.* Tampa, FL: American College of Physician Executives.

Sloan, S., and R. Fralicx. 2011. "Is There a Leader in the House?" *Hospitals & Health Networks Daily.* Published August 11. www.hhnmag.com/hhnmag/HHNDaily/HHNDailyDisplay.dhtml?id=4680008273.

Tuso, P. J. 2003. "The Physician as Leader." *The Permanente Journal* 7 (1): 68–72.

CHAPTER 5

Physicians in Management and Leadership Positions

Discussion heard at a healthcare conference:

A recent MD/MBA graduate: Good leadership is about realistic plans and strong controls.

Physician executive: No, I really disagree. I think that your wording is in error—management, not leadership, is about planning, organizing, and controlling.

Health system CEO: I certainly agree with that. Management concerns itself with the day-to-day and builds systems and controls that ensure continuity, reduce variance, and increase predictability. Leadership looks farther into the future and concerns itself with what changes need to be made to those systems to meet the changes that naturally occur in the environment.

Executive in charge of an employed-physician network: In some ways, I see this clearly in our network. My practice managers need to be practicing effective management so that our physicians are productive, we give high-quality care, we are run efficiently, and we pay attention to patient satisfaction. Yet a lot of my job is to anticipate future changes. For example, I am now studying some significant population moves in the southern section of our primary service area. If we don't get physician offices located there soon, our competitor will take market share from us.

Concluding comment from the recent MD/MBA graduate: So, organizations need both management and leadership.

An increasing number of jobs in healthcare organizations allow physicians to move out of clinical roles and assume administrative ones. Some jobs involve focused, day-to-day management, while others are more strategic and long range and focus on making changes in the future. An understanding of both of these types of roles is critical in establishing opportunities for putting physicians in jobs in which they have their hands on the levers and controls of organizations. In essence, physician managers steer the car, making immediate adjustments, while physicians in leadership roles plan the entire trip and consider detours and challenges in the road yet unseen. And many physicians wear both management and leadership hats.

This chapter discusses the differences between management and leadership and reviews the types of positions that physicians often move into. Understanding the differences is crucial when moving physicians into roles that affect the direction of the organization. Simply put, some physicians may not be well suited for positions that require a lot of leadership activity, but they may be excellent as managers.

John Kotter (2001), Harvard professor of management, suggests that "management promotes stability and copes with complexity, and leaders press for and cope with change. One is not better than the other, as both are necessary for success."

We hope the following general statements summarizing that conclusion might better present the case.

Management and leadership are different. This bears repeating—there is a difference between management and leadership. Yet most books and articles either (a) use the words interchangeably (as even we have done in some places in this book) or (b) portray management as bad and leadership as good. In this chapter, we strive to use the terms separately and distinctly. Moreover, we believe that both are positive.

Management is a core activity of running an organization. Management is a function and activity whereby individuals plan and organize work, projects, and operations. They use budgets, controls, and metrics and direct the work of others in achieving this work. Management is focused mostly on the immediate.

Leadership is future oriented. Leadership, on the other hand, is more abstract and focuses more on the future. The functions and activities of leadership pertain to developing needed change to meet the future. In his book *The Seven Habits of Highly Effective People*, Stephen Covey (1990) says, "Management is efficiency in climbing the ladder of success; leadership determines whether the ladder is leaning against the right wall."

Kotter (1996) states, "Management is a set of processes that can keep a complicated system of people and technology running smoothly. The most important aspects of management include planning, budgeting, organizing, staffing, control-

Exhibit 5.1: Leadership Versus Management

Leadership	Management
Strategic	Tactical
Concerned more with long term	Concerned more with short term
Typically focused on vision and strategy	Typically focused on production and service
Vision oriented	Task oriented
Strategically develops the plan	Executes the plan
Changes the status quo	Works with the status quo
Creativity important	Practicality important

ling, and problem solving. Leadership is a set of processes that creates organizations in the first place or adapts them to significantly changing circumstances. Leadership defines what the future should look like, aligns people with that vision, and inspires them to make it happen despite the obstacles."

Refer to Exhibit 5.1 for an illustration of the differences between management and leadership.

In the era of clinical integration, the role of the hospital-sponsored or health system–sponsored medical group requires a clear understanding of the differences between management and leadership. These differences are shown in more detail in Exhibit 5.2.

Management and Leadership

Readers should consider the roles that physicians might play in their organizations and apply the following statements to them:

1. Jobs may require (a) mostly management skills and behaviors and *few* leadership skills and behaviors, (b) mostly leadership skills and behaviors and *few* management skills and behaviors, or (c) both.
2. Some individuals excel at both management and leadership, while others excel primarily at one or the other. Organizations—and those in both management and leadership positions—would do well to understand this deeply and use great caution when hiring individuals in either role.

Exhibit 5.2: Defined Group Management and Leadership Positions

Board Chairperson (Physician)	Leads the Board
	◆ Serves as board spokesperson ◆ Establishes board agendas ◆ Oversees board committees and work products ◆ Works with the hospital-sponsored medical group (HSMG) president and hospital VP health group to define issues and policies for consideration by hospital and HSMG
HSMG President (Physician)	**Leads the HSMG/Physicians**
	◆ Leads and oversees the development of HSMG clinical policies ◆ Manages HSMG physician issues and concerns, including implementation of the physician compensation plan as approved by the board ◆ Supports the VP health group in the interaction and integration of HSMG and hospital policies and functions ◆ Manages the alignment of HSMG and hospital medical staff interfaces and, where appropriate, issue resolution
Hospital VP Health Group/Group Practice Administrator	**Leads HSMG Operations and Interfaces with Administrator**
	◆ Manages and oversees the daily operations of HSMG ◆ Manages the integration and alignment of hospital-sponsored services to the HSMG ◆ Manages the analysis of issues and policies for consideration by the HSMG chairperson, president, and board ◆ Manages financial accountability to the hospital

3. Typically, the higher a particular position is in an organization, the more that job demands leadership rather than management skills. But we do believe that individuals, no matter their level in an organization, frequently can and do exhibit *both* leadership and management skills and behaviors.
4. Educational programs, especially for physicians, often commingle management and leadership topics, which frequently creates confusion.

MANAGEMENT VERSUS LEADERSHIP

For the past 20 years, management and leadership literature has had more than its share of commentary that management is *bad* and that leadership is *good*, or that all should aspire toward gaining leadership positions. Many books suggest that one should strive to get out of the doldrums of management and step into the exciting world of leadership.

This plethora of communication labeling leadership and management in such a way has caused some problems for those in charge of organizations. The first is that the traditional areas of management have been given short shrift. The second is that there now seems to be a viewpoint that management and leadership are mutually exclusive. A person chooses to be one or the other, but cannot practice both. We vehemently disagree. Consider, for example, the following "day in the life" of a vice president of medical affairs:

7:00–8:30 a.m. Meet with the medical executive committee with a standard agenda of (a) approval of credentials, (b) hearing the architect's report on medical staff lounge renovations, and (c) hearing the routine pharmacy and therapeutics committee report (mostly management practiced during this time).

8:45–9:15 a.m. Review monthly calendar with administrative assistant and discuss new office arrangement (mostly management practiced during this time).

9:30–10:00 a.m. Meet with strategic planning consultant to review the backgrounds of the physician members of the strategy task force (both management and leadership practiced at this meeting).

10:00 a.m.–Noon. Meet with the strategic planning consultant to review the major changes in population shifts in the primary service area, the age distribution of primary care physicians in this geographical area, and the current practices that might be available for purchase in the area (mostly leadership practiced during this time).

Noon–1:30 p.m. Luncheon at the city club with retired members of the medical staff (both management and leadership practiced at this meeting).

5:00–7:00 p.m. Meet with the cardiology group, with whom the organization has a co-management agreement to discuss (a) opening additional satellite locations in two neighboring counties, (b) affiliating with a large primary care group practice, and (c) the backlog in the cath lab (both management and leadership practiced at this meeting).

Why is this distinction important? Why is it much more than a battle of semantics?

- Some physicians are adept and skilled at running an operating room or a cath lab. Much of what they do is day to day, tactical, and not at all strategic. Some of these physicians aspire to other positions, usually high in an organization, but are not skilled enough to effectively work at that level. Not every physician who can run the bed board in an OR is suited to be president of a health system.
- Some physicians are poorly placed (selected, elected, hired) in management or leadership positions. As an example, the group practice board chair getting involved in day-to-day staffing and hiring decisions in each practice location is detrimental to the organization.
- Some physicians move into positions to "fix" specific management problems (e.g., the family medicine physician who takes responsibility for billing and collections), and others move into positions to address leadership challenges (e.g., the physician concerned about the population health issues in the community). The two examples require different skills and behaviors. Properly matching skill sets with the demands of the job—whether leadership or management—is critical.
- The content of educational programs is different for management and leadership. Management education programs teach subjects such as budgeting, establishing management controls, and handling staffing issues. Leadership programs introduce topics on long-range strategic planning, forecasting, and building coalitions.

REVIEW OF DIFFERENT PHYSICIAN POSITIONS

The following descriptions of the comparative proportions of leadership and management core competencies needed for potential physician positions echo Covey's

(1990) comment that management is about climbing the ladder of success and leadership is about making sure the ladder is leaning against the right wall.

Physician CEO: A 75–25 match of leadership and management skills is required; the physician CEO needs to know both that the ladder is on the right wall and how to climb it.

Physician chief operations officer (COO): Requires 20 percent leadership skills and 80 percent management skills; the physician COO first and foremost needs to know how to climb the operational ladder.

Physician chief medical informatics officer (CMIO): Requires 40 percent leadership and 60 percent management; the physician CMIO needs to know that the medical informatics ladder is on the right wall, must constantly reevaluate that position, and, perhaps more important, must know how to climb the informatics ladder.

Physician chief quality officer (CQO): Surprisingly, the mix of core competencies has changed; the mix used to be 20 percent leadership and 80 percent management, but now it is 40–60. The physician CQO needs to know, in a changing quality landscape, that the quality ladder is on the right wall and that the wall may be changing. She also needs to be able to climb the ladder in an enterprise quality plan.

Physician chief medical officer (CMO): While the percentage mix depends greatly on the type of organization and the role the CMO plays, this position most likely requires a 50–50 mix of leadership and management core competencies. The physician CMO needs to know where the medical ladder is and that it is on the right wall; he also needs to know how to climb it in a variety of different circumstances. Typically, in larger organizations, the CMO will spend more time on leadership activities.

Physician VP for business development: Requires a 60–40 split of leadership and management core competencies; the key, again, is getting the business development job done.

Physician VP for managed care: Requires a similar 60–40 split.

Physician VP for strategy: Requires 80 percent leadership and 20 percent management; the physician VP for strategy needs to make sure the ladder is on the right strategic wall and that climbing it is an executable strategy.

Physician VP for managing employed physician networks: Even though employed physicians may not be in separate networks and network physicians may not be employed, the physician VP for managing employed physician networks needs a 60–40 mix of core competencies—60 percent is knowing the physician relations ladder is on the right wall and 40 percent is climbing it.

An important note is in order here. The selection of percentages may vary greatly from organization to organization; the key thought is that organizations understand the differences.

CONCLUSION

While this chapter addresses the differences between management and leadership, it also recognizes that these words are often used interchangeably. Further compounding the confusion is the existence of jobs that have both management and leadership demands and individuals who have both management and leadership skills and competencies. We strongly suggest that readers keep this important differentiation in mind as they continue reading.

Thoughts for Consideration

How did you define *management* before reading this chapter?

Has that definition changed?

How did you define *leadership* before reading this chapter?

Has that definition changed?

What kinds of management excellence have you seen physicians display?

What kinds of leadership excellence have you seen physicians display?

Which positions in your organization demand management skills?

Which positions in your organization demand leadership skills?

Does your organization have educational programs focused on matching the right skills—management or leadership—with the right position?

SUGGESTED READING

Dye, C. F. 2002. *Winning the Talent War: Ensuring Effective Leadership in Healthcare.* Chicago: Health Administration Press.

Dye, C. F., and A. N. Garman. 2006. *Exceptional Leadership: 16 Critical Competencies for Healthcare Leaders.* Chicago: Health Administration Press.

Kotter, J. P. 1999. *What Leaders Really Do.* Boston: Harvard Business Review Press.

————. 1990. *A Force for Change: How Leadership Differs from Management.* New York: Free Press.

Murray, A. 2009. "What Is the Difference Between Management and Leadership?" *Wall Street Journal.* Published April 7. http://guides.wsj.com/management/developing-a-leadership-style/what-is-the-difference-between-management-and-leadership/.

CHAPTER 6

The Vice President of Medical Affairs Position and Its Transition

While enjoying lunch at a recent industry conference, five vice presidents of medical affairs (VPMAs) discussed their jobs:

VPMA 1: I love what I am doing. I spend 50 percent of my time in patient care areas talking with other docs and nurses about quality and patient safety. I've also begun to show others how quality and utilization interrelate. The rest of the week I slot myself into hospitalist shifts and cover unassigned patients in the emergency department.

VPMA 2: Fascinating. I can't say that I spend much time at all doing anything in quality. That area reports to the chief nursing officer. I spend most of my time in business development and managed care. I focus a lot on how we can expand our service lines, and my chief financial officer and I are frequently meeting with insurers, especially since we started some pilot pay-for-performance programs.

VPMA 3: You two sure get into some interesting things. I just started my VPMA position a year ago. After practicing surgery for 35 years, I thought this would be a good way to wind down and still make a contribution. I spend most of my time in the medical staff lounge listening to day-to-day problems that many of our physicians raise with me.

VPMA 4: Well, I guess I am the oddball here. Our entire medical staff is now employed, and my challenges are trying to create a common culture and building systems that make us feel more like a multispecialty group practice. I also spend a lot of my time on physician compensation and merging smaller practices into larger ones.

VPMA 5: I guess my job is the most unusual of all. While I used to spend a lot of time handling many of the activities all of you describe, I have reached a point where I spend practically all of my time helping our CEO and board to craft strategy. Our physician issues are so critical that they play out in practically all of our strategic initiatives.

> The vice president of medical affairs (VPMA) position has typically been the entry point into administration for most physicians. It is also the one position that most organizations have if they have a full-time physician administrative position. The role differs greatly from organization to organization, especially when compared to the traditional top executive positions like chief financial officer (CFO) or chief nursing officer. Yet the job is important when considering physician leadership matters. One of the most critical steps organizations can take is to ensure that their VPMA positions are well defined.

THE VPMA: WHAT IS IT?

Interestingly, the VPMA often has more variation in roles, duties, responsibilities, and even titles than any other position on the senior executive team. VPMAs can be many things to an organization, and the differences, as shown in the opening vignette, represent the tip of the iceberg. Edward O'Connor and Marlena Fiol (2006) put it well: "The term 'physician executive' is simply a signpost—an indication that a physician is occupying an executive role. The actual definition of duties associated with the title varies greatly across organizations and positions."

Because a VPMA can be so many different things to an organization and to an executive team, defining the position clearly—specifying both roles and functions—is necessary. *Roles* are the expected social and interactive behaviors of an individual on a team. At times they are traditionally prescribed (e.g., the CFO is the "guardian" of the money; the human resources executive is the "people conscience" of the organization). Other times, they are tied to the style characteristics of an individual (e.g., implementer, father or mother figure, coach, nitpicker).

Following are some of the typical roles frequently played by a VPMA:

◆ **Advocate.** The VPMA often is asked to play an advocacy role—either for the medical staff or for the administration. Often, VPMAs are expected to bridge the gap between the physician perspective and the executive team.

◆ **Liaison.** Similar to the advocate role, the VPMA is viewed as the link between the medical staff and administration—an ambassador, if you will. Along with this role, the VPMA is often expected to play the role of messenger, bringing not-so-good news to either party.

♦ **Police officer.** Historically, VPMAs have played the lead role in peer review processes, risk management, and medical staff code-of-conduct matters. Those who play this role monitor and enforce policy.

♦ **Quality officer.** Many VPMAs essentially serve as chief quality officers for their organizations, spending most of their time monitoring quality and making needed interventions. The Institute of Medicine's *Crossing the Quality Chasm* (2001) and *To Err Is Human: Building a Safer Health System* (1999) made many VPMA/physician executives the champions in evidence-based medicine and quality improvement.

Functions, on the other hand, are more formally tied to a specific position and spell out major job components or a number of tasks that contribute to the accomplishment of an overall objective. Often listed in a job description, some typical functions of a VPMA position include the following:

♦ Managing the medical staff office
♦ Managing credentialing and privileging
♦ Leading clinical improvement
♦ Directing quality assurance
♦ Directing utilization review activities
♦ Mediating professional disputes and interdepartmental problems
♦ Managing the physician dispute-resolution process
♦ Recruiting physicians
♦ Managing the implementation of electronic health records
♦ Guiding physician leadership development and succession planning
♦ Supporting the hospital's continuing medical education program
♦ Ensuring that medical staff efforts meet the standards of accrediting bodies

Concerns

The role confusion, mixed expectations, and varied nature of the VPMA position can lead to significant concerns and problems with the position.

In organizations that still have a significant number of voluntary medical staff

♦ the VPMA may supplant the role and authority of the selected president of the medical staff;

- the VPMA may take too much of an advocacy role for one side or the other (pro administration or pro medical staff);
- the CEO may not want the VPMA to gain too much influence with the physicians and therefore may either overtly or covertly minimize the VPMA's influence or authority;
- the VPMA may be forced into an "enforcer" role—riding herd on bad utilization, poor quality, and recalcitrant physicians;
- if the VPMA is selected from within the medical staff, historical ties or allegiances to some physicians may cause political problems;
- the VPMA may be expected to "fix the doctor problem" (whatever that may be);
- the VPMA may have an unclear role; or
- the CEO, board, and executives may assume that the VPMA, as a physician, is broadly representative of how the entire physician collective thinks and operates.

In organizations that no longer have a significant number of voluntary medical staff or that have system roles without specific care units attached to them

- the VPMA position may be filled by an individual who does not comprehend the transition that is occurring in the industry and still clings to the "good old days" when doctors were part of a club-type culture, or
- the VPMA role itself may become an anachronism in that it has no clearly delineated role other than to deal with the (now declining) voluntary medical staff.

Title: CMO or VPMA?

Over the years, the question of using the VPMA title versus the chief medical officer (CMO) title has been raised. Dister (2009) concluded that "survey findings do not offer a definite answer to this question. Healthcare organizations and physician leaders widely vary in their readiness to put a stake in the ground on this subject." For the purposes of our discussions, we do not find any significant differences to warrant great discussion.

TRANSITION—TO WHAT?

The VPMA role is one that has experienced much transition and continues to do so. Among the reasons for these changes are the following:

- The demise of the voluntary medical staff. Historically, many VPMA positions were added as extenders, with the primary responsibility of providing support for elected medical staff officers.
- The growth in the number of employed physicians
- Increasing emphasis on patient safety and quality
- The development of in-house specialists, coupled with the decline of primary care physicians physically coming to the acute care hospital. Because the VPMA is often the only full-time administrative physician, giving her responsibility for areas such as hospitalists and intensivists or the employed physician network seems most logical.
- Adding traditional acute care operations departments. Some organizations have assigned administrative responsibility for departments such as pharmacy, radiology, lab, and others to the VPMA portfolio. As a result of these shifts, some VPMA positions have morphed into hospital COO jobs.
- The drive toward building alignment. The 1990s and the early potential move toward capitated reimbursement began some of the early shifts toward shared incentives. These initiatives served as the forerunner of clinical integration.

Many of the future developments that may occur with VPMA positions will be tied to three major changes occurring in the healthcare field: consolidation, the need for more clinical operations managers to deal with the transformation of the patient care system, and the development of clinical integration.

Consolidation. The industry has started to see significant consolidation, either through mergers and acquisitions or through various forms of affiliation. Experts posit that in the next five to ten years, the number of hospitals and health systems will significantly drop (Fields 2011). Although for some organizations this change may not occur for a few years, consolidation will likely lead to the ultimate elimination of the more traditional VPMA role. As organizations join larger organizations to gain the efficiencies of clinical integration, the jobs for full-time physician executives will be more clearly defined (e.g., manage the hospitalists, intensivists, and other in-house specialists; lead quality efforts; lead specific acute care business units). Consolidation will also create the need for physician leaders to help reorganize the physician practices into larger and more cohesive groups.

Transformation. An example of this new approach to systems improvement in organizations is described by Dr. Imran Andrabi (2012) of Mercy Health Partners, who indicated that his organization's efforts involved "bringing together a multidisciplinary group from all levels of the hospital to explore ways to make our processes more efficient." Whether labeled transformation, Lean, or some other name, those organizations in the forefront of these changes all indicate a great need for significant physician leadership. Much of it comes from the VPMA.

Clinical integration. Clinical integration will also give rise to specific new physician jobs and job titles. Clinical integration has many meanings, from simple activities designed around a specific disease (such as diabetes) to a full-fledged corporate mechanism designed to unite independent physicians and their hospital to focus on specific quality improvements within the entire health system. For some, the ultimate definition of clinical integration is a fully employed group of physicians who drive the entire care and quality process as a single group. We believe one of the better definitions is a simple one: Clinical integration is a form of organization that binds primary care physicians, physician specialists and subspecialists, and hospitals and health systems in a formal structure to work together to improve processes and outcomes using validated protocols, guidelines, and measures.

No matter the definition, clinical integration will give rise to more opportunities for the VPMA to transition in terms of roles, duties, and functions.

New titles. Today, three common titles exist for physician leaders: VPMA, CMO, and chief quality officer (CQO). In most organizations, the CMO and VPMA titles are interchangeable. But increasingly the CMO or VPMA has picked up traditional CQO responsibilities—or even supervises that position.

In the traditional hospital or health system environment, the VPMA (usually not called a CMO) was responsible for physician relations, the interface between the hospital and medical staff, and compliance with physician-oriented requirements of the hospital or health system's deeming organization (e.g., The Joint Commission, the Centers for Medicare & Medicaid Services). He often served as an ambassador, working to ensure that relationships remained positive among all parties. However, in the past several years, within a single hospital or health system, the VPMA or CMO has begun to gain responsibility for all things clinical, including the medical staff, quality initiatives, and physician strategy for both employed and independent providers. The newer role brings this top physician leader into more strategy development and, in many cases, business development. The more contemporary CMO or VPMA spends a great deal of time balancing the needs of independent and employed physicians because that position is generally responsible for all members of the medical staff. Indeed, one of the changes under clinical integration is that more executives carry the CMO title—a CMO, to many physicians, represents a broader function than just administration and is required to perform the clinical duties in a hospital environment.

More recently, hospitals and health systems have developed greatly expanded hospital-sponsored medical groups (HSMGs) or employed physician networks

(EPNs) and, for some, development of clinically integrated organizations (CIOs). As a result, the dynamic between the employed physicians in the HSMG or EPN and the independent physicians in private practice has grown more complex and comprehensive. Because the VPMA was largely responsible for inpatient activities of the medical staff, the term CMO has been used for a VPMA with expanded inpatient and outpatient physician management responsibilities. In other words, the CMO is responsible for all things clinical, including the medical staff, quality initiatives, and the organization's physician alignment strategy. The next-generation VPMA spends a great deal of time balancing the needs of independent and employed physicians in a CIO or value-based purchasing environment that considers the multiple needs of the many physician and nonphysician constituencies. As this clinical integration trend continues to expand, more executives will carry broader titles—in some cases, a CMO title, in other cases, an executive vice president. And, to many physicians, these titles represent a broader function and signify serving as a key member of the organization's senior leadership team.

A new position is emerging—the managing physician or president of the HSMG (the employed physicians or the EPN). That position is critically important because the HSMG is often the largest cost center in the hospital, and it is growing exponentially. As physicians integrate under an employment model, most of them lose money in a strict cost-accounting model on providing clinical services. This has become a flash point for many organizations, and understanding and managing those deficiencies are critical. The position is important as well because in a clinically integrated organization, the HSMG will be at the core of the physician component of what services the hospital and health system can offer.

Another emerging position is the chief medical information officer (CMIO). If that position is filled by a physician, and increasingly it is, that physician must learn to manage the interests of both the hospital and the physicians—employed, independent, and contracted. Ultimately, the CMIO is responsible for the management of all value-based plans, which must balance cost and quality. That is why a physician executive running the clinical information systems ideally should have both delivery system and payer expertise.

Operational Departmental Responsibilities

Many VPMAs are assigned specific operations departments. Historically, VPMAs would often have the medical library, continuing medical education (CME), and social services departments reporting to them. Over the past decade, though, the areas of operational responsibility for VPMAs have grown significantly. Some have been given direct line authority for acute care departments, such as radiology, pathology, and other clinical areas. Others have picked up line operations control over hospitalist programs, employed physician networks, and clinical integration entities. Still others are gaining executive authority over the implementation of the electronic medical record and other IT matters that relate to clinical areas. In the near future, seeing VPMAs morph into acute care executives in charge of entire clinical operations or heading up population health management matters would not be unusual.

KEY ISSUE IN HIRING A VPMA: INSIDER OR OUTSIDER?

One of the biggest issues facing many organizations with the VPMA position is the question of hiring from within the medical staff versus finding talent outside. Often, the decision to hire an internal candidate is influenced more by political considerations than by any other factors. For example, a popular physician within the medical staff may have aspired toward the position. Some organizations have even experienced campaign-like behavior from internal candidates who want the position. Tradition may have dictated that individuals move up through the ranks and eventually become the paid CMO. Turning to the outside may represent an insult to custom. Some organizations find that their medical staff leadership believes the CMO position is their position and, as a result, they should be the ones making the hiring decision. Many medical staff leaders believe in the "devil we know versus the devil we don't know" school of thought when it comes to selection decisions. The ability to have one of their own in the position is quite similar to the elected nature of the medical staff governing process. The following are the strongest arguments for hiring an internal candidate:

◆ Internal candidates know the local physician population better.
◆ Internal candidates have a better feel for the politics of the physician collective within the area.
◆ Internals have a better understanding of the managed care climate of the area.
◆ Internals have already established clinical credibility with the existing medical staff.
◆ The learning curve is much shorter for internal candidates.

Many organizations have hired a locally known and respected physician for their VPMA positions. Organizations often select an elder statesman who is nearing the end of his career and wants to wind down. The organization's leaders may feel that these internal candidates have served well and would therefore continue to be the best choice. Let there be no doubt: Many healthcare organizations have been well served by VPMAs who have come from within. Yet when selecting internal candidates, organizations frequently find that they perpetuate more traditional medical staff interventions as a result. The following points argue in favor of looking outside for a VPMA:

- Although lacking the local knowledge, external candidates often bring more creativity to the leadership process.
- The exposure that external candidates have had in other physician environments may enhance their understanding of alternative approaches to problems and strategic decisions.
- Much like the practices of benchmarking and best practices management, external VPMA candidates from other areas of the country and from other organizations bring new solutions, new approaches, and different views of strategy with them.
- Although not always the case, external candidates are often more dedicated to a career of physician leadership and are not as likely to be looking for a change of career or a way to wind down.
- External candidates enter an organization with no preconceived biases or political blocs to which they are indebted.

At times, the decision to go outside or stay inside hinges on the prescribed role of the VPMA. If the role is primarily intended to provide a more traditional interface between hospital administration and the medical staff, and to function more as an extension of the medical staff processes, then often an internal candidate is the better selection. However, if the VPMA is intended to serve in a broad operational and strategic executive role, then an individual with experiences in various locations may bring the most to the table.

In the final analysis, the decision should be made on the basis of which candidate can best meet the requirements of the job. If the role is more traditional (the liaison role), internals may actually be better suited for the position. If, however, the needs require more strategic leadership and a more active effort to lead change within the physician collective, externals will typically bring more value to the position.

A final consideration involves benchmarking internal candidates relative to those on the outside. Some organizations would be well served by introducing some externals into the interview and review process. Doing so can provide a stronger validation of the selection of the internal and eliminate the second-guessing that sometimes occurs as internal candidates make changes in their new position.

CONCLUSION

The massive changes now facing healthcare organizations will dictate changes in the VPMA position, its role, and its future. Organizations that still have large voluntary medical staffs will, in the near term, still need traditional VPMA support. Some organizations may even find themselves needing to create their first full-time VPMA positions. Others are finding their VPMA positions morphing into different roles. And in the near future, the VPMA position as the industry has known it for more than 60 years—the medical staff lounge ambassador—will disappear.

Thoughts for Consideration

Has your organization clearly delineated the role that your VPMA is to play?

Is that role based on how that position functioned in the past or on what the current and future healthcare environment demands?

Is the VPMA equal to other executives in your organization, with true authority and responsibilities?

Which typical VPMA role—advocate, liaison, police officer, or quality officer—does your institution need most?

Is your organization equipped to find and hire a VPMA who could, if needed, morph into a COO or CMO?

SUGGESTED READING

Linney, B. J. 2002. "VPMA = Very Busy Day: Physician Executive Faces Many Meetings, Critical Decisions in Typical Day." *The Physician Executive* 28 (2): 74–76.

O'Connor, E. J., and C. M. Fiol. 2006. "Reclaiming Physician Power: Your Role as a Physician Executive." *The Physician Executive* 32 (6): 46–50.

Tyler, J. L. 1999. "Vice President of Medical Affairs: Moving On Up to CEO? (The Evolving Role of the Physician Executive)." *The Physician Executive* 25 (5): 20–24.

Williams, S. J., and C. M. Ewell. 1997. "An Evolving Medical Leadership Position: Tomorrow's Vice President of Medical Affairs." *The Physician Executive* 23 (2): 16–20.

CHAPTER 7

The Transition to Leadership and Management

Comments to the physician making the transition to management:

"You've got to be kidding me."

"You have gone to the dark side. You've become one of them. You are now the enemy."

"You'll have a wider canvas."

"Why are you doing this? For another sentence in your obituary?"

"Great. Now we can get all our problems fixed."

"You are crazy."

"What a waste of training."

"Well, good luck—if that is *really* what you want to do."

Comments by the physician making the transition:

"I'm 50 years old, and I feel like I just got out of college."

"I'm probably in the highest-paid on-the-job training program in the world."

"This is not at all what I thought it would be."

"Career change—well, much more than that. I just cannot fully explain it."

"I wish I had done this sooner."

"Oh my, this is pretty scary."

One of the bigger changes in the life of a physician is the transition to a part-time or full-time management or leadership role. As a clear departure from the activities that compose the clinical practice of medicine, this new life requires significant change; for most, it causes a radical makeover. In some respects, it is much more than a simple career change. It requires a different outlook, a changed perspective, and new skills and competencies. And on top of all of this, as mentioned above in the opening comments, this switch can also lead to significant heckling and bewilderment from former colleagues. Physicians making these moves must be well prepared to manage the transition.

Put simply, moving from a clinical role to an administrative role is an enormous step for any physician—it represents a career change, a transition, a different job with different skill sets. And it requires adjustment, conversion, new thinking, and novel approaches to issues and problems. Physicians contemplating this change would be wise to consider the points this chapter raises. And those who are counseling or coaching physicians should ensure that these factors are given due consideration. A full awareness of the likely changes is important to keep in mind before venturing into any type of physician leadership development.

KEY ISSUES INVOLVED IN THE TRANSITION

Motivation

Many questions surface for physicians who are considering a move into administrative roles. But the central question is the simple "why?" (See "Tips on Making Career Changes.")

Dr. Martin Merry (1996) raises the following questions that should be considered before making the transition:

◆ Do I want to help create a better future for my practice, my patients, the profession, and healthcare generally, or am I just burned out and looking for something different?

- Do I possess (or am I willing to obtain) the core skills and traits that health-care leaders need?
- Am I willing to set aside past struggles with hospitals and insurance companies to work within a larger system for the good of healthcare generally?
- Am I ready to take the risks of leading change—including making errors, learning from successes and mistakes, and changing course (both personally and organizationally) as necessary?
- Do I have (or am I willing and able to develop) a sense of mission and vision that will enable me to think globally and act locally?
- We would add, "To what extent is there a comfort level in having patient care issues intertwined with business and strategic issues?" and "How comfortable is the physician leader in dealing with the gaps and conflicts between values and reality?"

Tips on Making Career Changes

- Explore the "why" of a career change first.
- Connect with someone who is already in the position.
- Define the positives and negatives of the change.
- Explore family support or reticence for the change.
- Try to shadow someone who is doing the job.
- Create an inventory of needed skills and competencies, and see where you compare.
- Write a narrative of what you plan to do, and ask others to review it.
- Be sure of your reasons—explore the "why" in greater detail.

Continuing to Practice

Because the entry point into administration is part-time for many physicians, the issue of practice should be addressed. Several themes arise for those physicians who consider continuing clinical practice while serving in an administrative position:

- Am I continuing to practice to provide a safety net if the administrative position does not work out?
- Am I practicing to garner the (clinical) respect of colleagues (if I do not practice, they will say, "You are no longer a doctor")?

- Am I practicing so that I can better identify the issues that practicing physicians face (e.g., system problems, organizational inefficiencies)?
- Is my reason for practicing more personal (e.g., to continue to maintain my sense of worth, or to keep contact with patients with whom I have relationships)?

A significant issue with practice for administrative physicians is identity. Physicians, perhaps more than other professionals, gain their identity from what they do. If asked what they do, nonphysician executives often answer by telling the questioner where they work ("I work at Capital City Health System") while physicians most often answer, "I am a doctor." The practice of medicine is very formal, whether because of the Hippocratic Oath, the status that society affords physicians, or the role that the physician takes on in the valued duty of caring for patients. Even the "white coat ceremony"—marking the transition into medical school and the welcome into the role of caring for patients—holds solemn meaning. The speeches that surround these events carry such words as *legacy, honor,* and *milestone.* These factors may make it more difficult for physicians to make the transition into leadership.

Some hospitals prefer to have physician executives who continue some type of practice. The reality, though, is that the stress and time demands of the position often prevent the physician from doing any kind of practice. Obviously, this may depend on the specialty and the type of organization. As the number of physician leadership opportunities grows in the complex world of clinical integration, there may be *fewer* chances for physician leaders to practice clinically.

Finally, many administrative physicians continue to practice because of organizational finances. While this is truer of smaller organizations that have more difficulty affording the salary of a full-time physician executive, some organizations provide part of the compensation and expect the physician to make up the rest through continuing clinical practice. While the authors are aware of many successful examples of this arrangement, some caution is necessary, especially going forward in the new integrated world, in continuing these types of situations.

One note of caution is in order regarding the time commitment that managing requires. The hours required of leaders and managers, physician or nonphysician, are long and often underestimated by physicians moving into administration positions. Also, the control of one's time is not as great when in a management or leadership position. Physicians practicing clinically have office hours, their patients come to them, and much of what they need is provided for them at the care site; the practice of clinical medicine has a certain routine to it. The opposite is true of administrative roles—unexpected events disrupt the time flow, data gathering is often scattered over several days, and the coordination of people and events is often totally out of the control of the executive. One physician executive commented that the biggest difference he experienced in his transition was the "tyranny of meetings and the calendar." Time management is often the single greatest challenge for new physician executives.

CHANGES YOU MAY NOT INITIALLY NOTICE

Some of the little changes that occur when moving into management and leadership often add up and create significant stress for physicians. Some may go unnoticed at first, while others hit physicians head-on. An awareness of these issues can make them less traumatic (see "Addressing the Issues of Continuing Practice").

Your performance is not just about you. After moving into leadership positions, physicians will see that they are evaluated more on organizational measures of success than on individual factors. Executive performance evaluation systems usually track financials and budgets, aggregate quality indicators, patient satisfaction scores, and human resources engagement scores. Performance in these areas is affected by many people. Physicians who have for years competed on an individual basis may find this a rude awakening.

What are you first? Physicians who make the transition often find an internal psychological confrontation regarding their identity. Are they physicians first and leaders second, or vice versa? While this may not seem to be a significant point, it can cause great personal conflict. This is particularly true when a decision has to be made that relates to clinical practice or areas that nonphysicians typically have little authority over.

You are not a real doctor any longer. Although this sentiment is often not expressed out loud by others, physicians who move into leadership roles report feeling this and having some distress as a result.

You are now the "hospital" or the "health system" or "administration" and therefore the enemy. Physicians making the transition report significant challenges in dealing with the perception that they have moved to some other side or point of view ("You are now a suit"). This can cause great emotional upheaval and is a factor that needs to be confronted.

You are engaged, but other physicians are not. A Gallup study reported that of more than 6,000 physicians surveyed, only 10 percent were fully engaged with their hospital, while 42 percent were actively disengaged (Paller 2005). According to aggregate results from nationwide physician engagement surveys done by Morehead Associates (Morton 2011), "Physicians are still struggling to connect with, and gain confidence in, hospital administration." The study concluded that physicians' lowest scores were reflected in their confidence in their health system or hospital. This realization can often cause physician leaders to question their move into leadership or, worse, their effectiveness in leadership.

> **Addressing the Issues of Continuing Practice**
>
> - Be seen in clinical settings. Make a weekly habit of spending a concentrated amount of time in some area of practice.
> - Read and stay current on clinical trends.
> - Maintain board certification.
> - Play a role in medical education (teach or precept), even if peripherally.
> - Stay active and engaged in the organization's quality review and improvement programs.

Emotions run high in this job. Interestingly, the Gallup study (Paller 2005) also reported significant findings that even though physicians are scientific in their approach to the practice of medicine ("Decisions are driven by two distinct thought patterns—rational and emotional. Physicians use rational thinking all the time"), they become quite emotional when making decisions that relate to the hospitals where they practice or other business matters.

PREPARING FOR THE TRANSITION EDUCATIONALLY

Physician leaders and managers need education in leadership and management. Noting the great complexity of the healthcare business and industry is critical. As Peter Drucker (1973) commented, "The hospital is one of the most complex social institutions around." Many physicians have found that getting an additional degree (e.g., a master's in business administration, public health, or health administration) provides knowledge that helps with the transition into administrative medicine. "All physicians need some kind of business training," states Maria Y. Chandler, a pediatrician with an MBA who is an associate clinical professor in the medical and business schools at the University of California, Irvine (Freudenheim 2011).

While much of leadership requires competencies that can be learned and practiced in any field, many aspects of health system management require specialized knowledge in subjects such as finance, administration, law, human resources, information technology, and operations. Moreover, experience in these subjects is also required. Learning needs to be coupled with exposure and experience—in management, in leadership.

On the other hand, an individual with an advanced management degree is not necessarily competent to perform. Experts say that an MBA will not necessarily help physicians run their practices better or help them earn more money. But it can be a necessary step for the physician on a trajectory toward an executive position with a hospital or health system (Routson 2011). One physician executive commented, "My master's degree may not have changed all of my approaches to issues, but it did give me new perspective and broadened my point of view."

A major consideration in selecting a master's program is determining whether to select a "pure" business-related MBA or a master's program specifically geared toward healthcare professionals. There is no simple answer, but consideration should be given to the time commitment required, the content area(s) where the physician may feel some deficiency, the cost, and degree of management and leadership experience that the physician already has.

CONCLUSION

The best way to describe the transition from the clinical practice of medicine to the practice of management or leadership is with words such as *major, momentous, epic,* or *significant.* Physicians making the change would be wise to seriously consider the pros and cons. Those decision makers who bring full-time clinicians into administrative roles should also gain a deeper understanding of the issues faced.

Thoughts for Consideration

How many of the comments in the opening section of this chapter have you heard?

Does your organization offer adequate training resources for physicians moving into executive leadership?

Does your organization have someone who can discuss the role, functions, typical duties, rewards, and other aspects of physician executive positions?

Is your physician leadership selection process sensitive to the personal issues faced by physicians moving into these positions?

(continued)

Can your organization integrate various levels of continued clinical practice by physicians moving into leadership positions?

Do you adequately prepare physicians for the culture shock of leaving clinical practice for executive leadership?

SUGGESTED READING

Avakian, L. 2010. *Helping Physicians Become Great Managers and Leaders.* Chicago: AHA Press.

Babitsky, S., and J. J. Mangraviti. 2009. *Non-Clinical Careers for Physicians.* Falmouth, MA: SEAK Inc.

Balik, B. M., and J. A. Gilbert. 2010. *The Heart of Leadership: Inspiration and Practical Guidance for Transforming Your Health Care Organization.* Chicago: AHA Press.

Fernandez, R. 2010. *Physicians in Transition: Doctors Who Successfully Reinvented Themselves.* Fort Collins, CO: 50 Interviews Inc.

McKenna, M. K., and P. A. Pugno. 2005. *Physicians as Leaders: Who, How and Why Now?* London: Radcliffe Publishing.

Nankervis, C. 2003. "Choosing Between Clinical Practice and Administration." *Family Practice Management.* Accessed October 5, 2012. www.aafp.org/fpm/2003/0100/p39.html.

Urman, R. D., and J. M. Ehrenfeld. 2012. *Physicians' Pathways to Non-Traditional Careers and Leadership Opportunities.* New York: Springer Publishing.

CHAPTER 8

Covering the Basics

Physicians believe the prime contributing factors to improving relationships between themselves and hospitals are administrative responsiveness to physician concerns and participation in operational decisions—both grounded in ongoing communication.

—Roger A. Hughes, 2005

The way I see it, a lot of healthcare organizations get into trouble spending lots of time and money on elaborate physician leadership programs when they don't even do the basics well at all. And I am just not sure they really care.

—Anonymous CEO, May 21, 2012

When training physician leaders, many organizations gloss over the basics. Yet those who engage in sports, music, or other pursuits realize the applicability of the fundamentals. Handling complexity requires a foundation in the essentials. The authors suggest that this chapter be used as an "audit checklist," a way for readers to do a quick assessment of their efforts in building physician support and collaboration, which ultimately will enhance physician leadership and involvement.

While many of the suggestions raised in this chapter may seem straightforward or simplistic, readers must realize that the nitty-gritty of relationships is critical. Before moving on to the next chapter, readers would be wise to carefully consider their approaches—and successes—with these and similar approaches to building connections and bonds with physicians. This chapter is

(continued)

> critical because working with physicians by definition involves so many complex factors. There are conflicts and dysfunctional physicians, the issue of organizational structure, and the fundamental need to address communications. For our readers who may not have all the fundamentals in place to deal with physicians, this might be a good kick-off chapter. These are the basics.

PHYSICIAN COMMUNICATIONS

Our chapter begins with a basic examination of communications—the element that is typically blamed for the majority of organizational ills. Many satisfaction surveys, particularly those with physicians, suggest that communications can be improved; in fact, many surveys reviewed by the authors showed that physician satisfaction levels with communications were usually lower than satisfaction levels of employees in other healthcare organizations. Addressing effective communications in great detail is beyond the scope of this book, but we offer the following points regarding communications with physicians.

Use surveys. Organizations that have the greatest success with their physician communication programs use various surveying techniques. Surveys can be in-depth and formalized (usually done every two to three years), or they can be simpler and shorter. Either option can provide ample data about physician views and thoughts. Dr. Lee Hammerling of ProMedica Health occasionally uses postcard surveys with three or four simple questions to gain a quick gauge on specific issues. When the issues are complex, however, some organizations use focus groups to capture more comprehensive information about physician opinions.

Morehead, a survey research firm that conducts physician satisfaction surveys, reports that its "highest-scoring physician engagement survey items in 2010 were related to physicians' confidence in the nursing staff" (Morton 2011). Yet, the lowest scores on their surveys related to their confidence in administration. Moreover, an important area addressed whether or not physicians felt they had adequate input into decisions that affect them and if hospital administration was responsive to their feedback. Surveys are excellent tools to capture a lot of data and minimize the chance of overreacting to issues that are only concerning a few physicians.

Use one-on-one communication. The best communications with physicians are usually individualized and personal. Group communications often fail, likely for several reasons:

◆ Emphasis on individual relationships. Physicians typically focus more on relationships than executives do, meaning their communication styles are developed on a one-on-one basis. This is the nature of working with patients. Executives, on the other hand, generally communicate facts, strategy, and concepts to groups of people.

♦ Communicating about feelings less than facts. In their training, physicians focus on the care of individuals, and this typically plays a significant role in the development of their communication style. Conversations with patients begin with feelings and an assessment of well-being. Even though physicians deal with quantitative measures in patient care (e.g., temperature, blood pressure, pulse), interactions with patients also involve qualitative matters, such as emotions and hope.

♦ Communications rich with listening. Physicians are typically good listeners in the clinical setting. To be effective clinicians, physicians must listen intently and comprehend more than just what is being said. This style is often opposite that of many executives, who, although charged with the need for good listening skills, often spend more time giving commands and directives.

To improve communication with physicians, meet physicians one-on-one whenever possible, build personal relationships that enhance the nature of one-on-one communications, and develop more intimate communication approaches, such as seeing physicians in smaller social settings or in more relaxed settings than the office. Although e-mail may be a more efficient form of communication, a face-to-face chat will provide better results when trying to build and maintain relationships.

Use the scientific method. Physicians learn through questioning and by using data in a scientific manner. Executives deal with great subjectivity, especially when considering more of their time is devoted to leadership activities, dealing with diverse personalities, and developing strategy (which by its nature is *not* quantitative).

When communicating with physicians, use data as much as possible and allow physicians the opportunity to question and challenge.

Examine the foundation of your communication. Executives use their position or status as the focal point of their communications, while physicians use their clinical knowledge and skills. Try to get physicians to see you (the executive) as a *person* rather than an *office* (the president or COO or VPMA).

Change the location of communication. Many successful executives have learned that going to the physical location where physicians engage in their clinical activity enhances communication. These executives use their physician relations staff to expand the number of physicians with whom they can make contact at their office locations. Similarly, many organizations realize the influence that office managers have with their physicians and try to develop opportunities to engage them in communication.

Spread the duties of communication. Many executives fail to realize that leaders other than themselves can take responsibility for communications. The following strategies can help executives share communication responsibilities with others:

- Assign other executives responsibility for specific key physicians so that more personalized and frequent communications can take place.
- Be certain that physicians understand the lines of communications within larger hospitals or health systems.
- Ensure that when physician practices are acquired and those physicians become employees of the larger hospital or health system, communications do not fall through the cracks. A heavier focus than usual may be critical during this time to ensure a successful transition.
- Ensure that physicians know they have an advocate who will always champion their viewpoints. This function may be one of the more important for the physician relations staff.

Identify and reduce the barriers to effective communications. Communication is often complicated by the complex relationships that exist in a professional setting. Working with physicians requires that special attention be paid to the following possible barriers:

- The choice of words executives use influences communications. Obviously, misinterpretation and distortion of meaning can cause tension.
- Defensiveness, past problems, and nonverbal forms of communication such as tone may stress relationships with physicians.
- Unreliable or inconsistent messages can lead to communications issues.
- Executives who are hesitant to be candid with physicians may create a difficult environment.
- Perceptual biases—and those often caused by incorrect or incomplete data— frequently create the biggest problems between nonphysician executives and physicians.
- Believing stereotypes about certain physicians (e.g., surgeons just want to cut to the issue; some specialties are motivated only by money; pathologists want to study the issue) creates true barriers to effective communications.
- How we perceive communications is greatly affected by the experiences we have had with the individuals doing the communicating.

Managing meetings. Meeting management may create some of the most profound communications concerns for physicians. Well-recognized meeting management skills are often overlooked by executives; moreover, the realization that meetings are expensive activities for physicians (even employed ones) suggests that executives do not take them very seriously. Remember that most physicians earn their paycheck from seeing patients, not from administrative duties.

Some simple suggestions for more effective meetings are:

- Be clear about the purpose of meetings. Is the meeting strategic or tactical? Will the result be a decision? Is the meeting designed to generate ideas? Is it a "show-and-tell" meeting to get status reports? Is it designed to communicate some item of interest?
- Start and end on time, and follow basic rules of courtesy—no electronic grazing.
- Avoid drift. If a participant deviates from the topic at hand, get that person back to it. If an argument starts, call the people on it and get refocused.
- Be prepared to tell people if they are talking too much.
- Encourage group discussion to get all points of view and ideas.
- Set an amount of time for each item on the agenda. If discussion increases on a topic past the allotted time, ask if further time is really necessary.
- Be very specific about the action items—who has agreed to do what and by when? At the meeting's end, review these items so they are crystal clear to everyone.
- Follow up by e-mail.
- Meetings should stay tightly focused. Any item that can be resolved between two people should be moved offline.
- Conduct a periodic evaluation of meetings.

PHYSICIAN CONFLICT MANAGEMENT

General conflict management with physicians is a primary area of concern and is often managed poorly. Consider the following challenges that make these situations most difficult.

Issues with Physician Conflict

Failure to confront and manage conflict. As mentioned in the previous section, many executives are hesitant, often afraid, to raise conflict issues with physicians. Whether caused by concern with a high revenue generator for the organization or simply the fear of a volatile physician, this failure can lead to built-up tensions and result in explosive battles that can do more damage. Managing conflict is tough for physicians as well. "Physicians tend to be compulsive, perfectionistic, guilt-prone, with an exaggerated sense of responsibility, limited emotional expressiveness (especially with respect to anger), and significant communications deficits, in particular an inability to ask for help" (Andrew 1999).

Physicians who guard against revealing emotions. Conflict by its nature is often emotional, and physicians are trained to distance themselves from emotional issues involving their patients. When confronted by a conflict, physicians are often unaware of how to manage their emotions.

Reality versus perceptions. Physicians are normally trained to work with facts (reality) in their clinical work and not rely upon their perceptions. However, physicians often jump to conclusions in nonclinical situations when they do not have facts, and as a result, their perceptions may not reflect reality. This can cause significant problems, especially when trying to compete in the heat of conflict.

Facts versus compromise. The training and work of physicians are driven by fact-gathering, such as with a history and physical. This approach is not common to the negotiations that drive conflict management. Most conflicts get solved by some form of compromise, which is certainly *not* the solution to a patient care problem.

Lack of training in collaboration. Physician training is top-down and driven by a higher authority. In contrast, executive education places a heavy emphasis on teamwork and collaborative solutions. Only recently have medical schools and residency programs started training on team care.

Physician to Physician

Nothing replaces the ability to get to know physicians on a personal and more intimate basis. This exercise of time will go a long way toward reducing misunderstandings and conflict situations.
—Jacque Sokolov, MD

A final word is in order regarding those organizations that have a mix of employed and independent physicians. Organizations should recognize that this situation creates many conflicts. Independent physicians often feel that employed physicians are receiving greater benefits and that they are favored by the employing entity. This situation can cause conflict, especially when organizations are making a transition toward greater numbers of employed physicians. Those who have navigated these waters most successfully believe that the best approach is an open one in which discussions are held about the two groups of physicians, and concerns are addressed in a transparent manner.

DISRUPTIVE PHYSICIANS

One of the more significant challenges is the disruptive physician. The American Medical Association (2009) defines disruptive behavior in physicians as

> a style of interaction by physicians with others, including hospital personnel, patients and family members, that interferes with patient care or adversely affects the healthcare team's ability to work effectively. It encompasses behavior that adversely affects morale, focus and concentration, collaboration and communications and information transfer, all of which can lead to substandard patient care.

In 2009, The Joint Commission adopted a leadership standard (Leadership Standard LD.03.01.01) that requires accredited organizations to adopt and implement a code of conduct that defines and addresses disruptive behavior. The disruptive behavior policies should now include the following (Joint Commission 2009, 2008; Maruca 2009):

- Zero tolerance for intimidating and/or disruptive behaviors, especially criminal acts such as assault
- Concepts that address intimidating behaviors of physicians that are complementary and supportive of policies aimed at nonphysician staff
- Provisions that protect those individuals who report intimidating behaviors
- Methods of responding to patients and/or families who witness such behaviors
- Specifics regarding how and when to begin disciplinary action

Many factors in the current healthcare environment can increase the possibility of frustration and disruptive behavior by physicians. These include the enormous changes anticipated by health reform legislation; continuing managed care pressures; the increased number of physicians becoming employed by so-called large, impersonal corporations; productivity demands on employed physicians; increasing malpractice threats; patient challenges; and the continued favoritism of some physicians over others by hospitals and health systems. In the words of one physician, "It's just not as rewarding as it used to be to practice medicine."

Despite the new emphasis on addressing disruptive physicians and the code of conduct interventions, some physicians need more significant assistance, often because of substance abuse or severe anger-management challenges. We would encourage all leaders to become familiar with one or more of the physician support programs that are offered in the industry. Three of the better ones are the Comprehensive Assessment Program at Vanderbilt University (www.mc.vanderbilt.edu/root/vumc.php?site=vcap); the PACE Program at the University of California, San Diego (www.paceprogram.ucsd.edu/); and the Anderson and Anderson Anger Management programs at the University of California, Los Angeles (www.anderson services.com).

PHYSICIAN RELATIONS

Physician relations can be summed up simply: Organizations must know and understand what physicians want and need. Often called "satisfiers" or "physician drivers," these elements within an organization create either negative or positive feelings. Physician satisfiers can either help retain physicians as partners or create a revolving door with high turnover. Identifying and addressing these satisfiers is a critical aspect of physician leadership that often falls to physicians who are in management and leadership positions.

> I think one of the biggest problems is understanding the chain of command for physicians and knowing who is in charge. Unless there is a clear organizational flowchart for addressing the medical and nonmedical needs of the medical practices, there are problems.
> —*Bob Uslander, MD, founder of Doctors on Purpose (Gamble 2011)*

Highly effective organizations do not view this as giving physicians all that they ask for but instead see it as dealing with the daily irritants and roadblocks to effective delivery of patient care. Addressing these matters is simple. It involves paying attention to physicians and ensuring they have ample opportunities to express their desires and concerns. Most leaders who are effective in these areas typically spend significant amounts of time interacting with physicians. Christina Roman (2011) writes, "Hospital leaders with the best results all say the same thing: Get to know your doctors on a personal level." Ted Townsend, CEO of St. Luke's Hospital in Cedar Rapids, Iowa, said that "the best hospitals are finding ways to not just align incentives, but to build strong cultures of mutual respect for each other as the best place to start the focus on achieving best practices" (Gamble 2012).

What do physicians want most? We believe that most readers would recognize the following:

- Focus and emphasis on quality and patient safety, strong nursing staff, and supportive ancillary departments
- Respect and responsiveness (Some physicians say, "Many administrators simply do not know me.")
- Ease of work when practicing in the hospital (including easy parking and building access as well as access to supplies and equipment)
- Opportunity to access decision makers
- Input or involvement in management decision making
- Assurance that the rules apply to all
- Individualized support and help with electronic medical records
- Recognition and appreciation for what they do. Like all other people, physicians do like to be appreciated.
- Efficiency and respect for time

Physician Stress

A final consideration for physician satisfiers is how organizations deal with physician stress and behavioral issues, such as substance abuse and well-being. Medicine is a high-stress occupation. Consider the following statement from a physician describing his first shift as a doctor (Anderson 2009):

> Suddenly, the responsibility was mine. I inherited 25 patients to look after and I had to cope with the fear, the anxiety, and responsibility of trying as best I could to make them all better and get them home. And try I did, but here's the thing—the work never ends. One patient gets well enough to leave and within minutes, there'll be a new patient in the bed that's just been vacated.

> Tired of clawing through the bureaucracy of today's healthcare system just to break even, many physicians are opting to enter a hospital's fold so they can focus on medicine and maintain some semblance of work–life balance.
> —*Elyas Bakhtiari, 2008*

According to Bogue and colleagues (2006), "Physician stress can lead to career dissatisfaction, disruptive behavior, burnout and career exit, substance abuse, health concerns, personal and family problems, and in the worst cases, suicide." Riley (2004) provides additional insight into the various sources of stress for physicians. "Doctors consistently experience high intensity of work, conflicting time demands, and heavy professional responsibility, often in systems where physical and social resources are deficient, and there is the ever-present threat of medicolegal action. Further, doctors often have limited power to alter the conditions under which they work," he writes.

Leaders must recognize the special requirements of addressing physician well-being. One excellent example is the Mayo Clinic Department of Medicine Program on Physician Well-Being, which was created to promote physician well-being "through research, education, and the development of wellness promotion programs that foster physician satisfaction and performance" (Mayo Clinic 2012).

According to its website, "The program is dedicated to

- understanding and promoting physician well-being
- providing resources for physicians that help them promote their own wellness
- discovering personal and organizational approaches to prevent physician distress
- creating a workplace that is a source not only of energy expenditure but also energy renewal"

Physician Compact

One avenue toward better physician relations is the use of a physician compact. A compact is simply an agreement that provides specific guidance in the relationships between physicians and the larger organization (hospital, health system). There is a quid pro quo or reciprocal set of commitments and responsibilities for both parties. The process of developing a compact should be a joint exercise and involve representatives of both parties. In many ways, a compact can be considered a "psychological contract" describing the mutual duties, obligations, and viewpoints that exist between employers and employees.

Exhibit 8.1 shows an example of a compact created by Virginia Mason Medical Center in Seattle, Washington.

Is a written compact required? Not necessarily. What is important is the process—both sides should be ready to sit as equal parties to discuss and agree on common visions, goals, and obligations to one another. Much like a marriage, the compact represents a balance, a willingness to compromise, and a desire to uphold the greater good.

> Last week, someone asked me what our top performing administrators and senior leaders are doing to ensure their physicians are engaged. My response was that like a lot of things in life, most of it comes down to improving communication, building trust, and creating partnerships.
> —Brad Morton, 2011

Exhibit 8.1: Virginia Mason Medical Center Physician Compact

VIRGINIA MASON MEDICAL CENTER PHYSICIAN COMPACT

Organization's Responsibilities

Foster Excellence
- Recruit and retain superior physicians and staff
- Support career development and professional satisfaction
- Acknowledge contributions to patient care and the organization
- Create opportunities to participate in or support research

Listen and Communicate
- Share information regarding strategic intent, organizational priorities and business decisions
- Offer opportunities for constructive dialogue
- Provide regular, written evaluation and feedback

Educate
- Support and facilitate teaching, GME and CME
- Provide information and tools necessary to improve practice

Reward
- Provide clear compensation with internal and market consistency, aligned with organizational goals
- Create an environment that supports teams and individuals

Lead
- Manage and lead organization with integrity and accountability

Physician's Responsibilities

Focus on Patients
- Practice state of the art, quality medicine
- Encourage patient involvement in care and treatment decisions
- Achieve and maintain optimal patient access
- Insist on seamless service

Collaborate on Care Delivery
- Include staff, physicians, and management on team
- Treat all members with respect
- Demonstrate the highest levels of ethical and professional conduct
- Behave in a manner consistent with group goals
- Participate in or support teaching

Listen and Communicate
- Communicate clinical information in clear, timely manner
- Request information, resources needed to provide care consistent with VM goals
- Provide and accept feedback

Take Ownership
- Implement VM-accepted clinical standards of care
- Participate in and support group decisions
- Focus on the economic aspects of our practice

Change
- Embrace innovation and continuous improvement
- Participate in necessary organizational change

© 2001 Virginia Mason Medical Center

TEAM MEDICINE™

VIRGINIA MASON

SOURCE: Virginia Mason Medical Center (2001). Used with permission.

CONCLUSION

Maintaining relationships through effective communication and strong conflict-management approaches may be the critical link to effective physician leadership. Ensuring that the special needs of stressed physicians are addressed is vital, as is creating an environment that allows leadership to be most effective. Readers are cautioned to not view these practices as too simple and straightforward. Even though these elements are called *basics*, they serve as a solid foundation to more effective organizations. Any physician leadership program will have these areas covered both in terms of development and in organizational practices that enhance physician relations.

Thoughts for Consideration

Do your communication approaches with physicians recognize the special personalized nature of physician communication styles?

Do you use multiple techniques to ensure effective communications (spot surveys, town hall meetings, meetings with physicians in their office settings, seeing physicians in the lounge, using social media)?

Does your organization have an adequate rounding program to ensure that contact is made with multiple physicians and not just those who sit on organizational committees?

Is conflict with physicians and its appropriate management something avoided or embraced?

How many of the issues addressed in the Virginia Mason compact has your organization specifically addressed? Do you think the creation of a formal document such as a compact is necessary to gain the benefits of one?

Can you name the key physician satisfiers at your organization?

SUGGESTED READING

Bogue, R. J., J. G. Guarneri, M. Reed, K. Bradley, and J. Hughes. 2006. "Secrets of Physician Satisfaction." *The Physician Executive* 32 (6): 30–39.

Dawson, R. 2000. *Secrets of Power Negotiating*. Pompton Plains, NJ: Career Press.

Gabbard, G. O., and R. W. Menninger. 1989. "The Psychology of Postponement in the Medical Marriage." *Journal of the American Medical Association* 261 (16): 2378–81.

Katz, N. H., J. W. Lawyer, and M. Sweedler. 2010. *Communication and Conflict Resolution Skills*. Dubuque, IA: Kendall Hunt Publishing.

Patmas, M. A. 2012. "Physician Integration: Building Sustainable Networks in Integrated Health Systems." *The Physician Executive* 38 (1): 26–29.

Pfifferling, J. H. 1999. "The Disruptive Physician: A Quality of Professional Life Factor." *The Physician Executive* 25 (2): 56–61.

Silversin, J., and M. J. Kornacki. 2000. "Creating a Physician Compact That Drives Group Success." *Medical Group Management Journal* 47 (3): 54–62.

Part III

FUTURE STEPS

CHAPTER 9

The Changing Healthcare Environment and the Clinical Integration Imperative

Hospital Executive A: Am I a dinosaur? Does anyone else remember the days when running a hospital meant getting as many patients as possible through your doors and providing as many services as possible to each one?

Hospital Executive B: Oh, I remember. But it seems like we've been moving away from that for 25 years at least, starting with managed care, diagnosis-related groups, and then managed competition and integrated delivery systems. So why does it seem more urgent now than it has in the past?

Hospital Executive A: Exactly. It hasn't been business as usual for decades. But it feels like the pressure to integrate our clinical services and promise value to our payers has never been greater.

Hospital Executive B: It sure does. I suppose that poses two questions. First, why is that? And second, what do we do about it?

In the new world of healthcare reform, physician engagement and the clinical model—a balance of care delivery drivers, changing reimbursement, and meeting a growing number of quality metrics and requirements—will guide everything. Rigorous business planning and financial modeling will be required, and they must support payment methodologies used by health plan payers and the Centers for Medicare & Medicaid Services (CMS). Knowing the rules of how funds flow through health plans, clinically integrated organizations (CIOs), and accountable care organizations (ACOs)—and being able to model those rules specifically for your organization and potential value-based purchasing participation—will be essential. All aspects of physician leadership will be shaped by these factors.

A PRIMER ON CLINICAL INTEGRATION

Clinical integration has many definitions. They include the broad definition from Blue Consulting Services (2012), which describes it as "a myriad of efforts that have been made to coordinate, or integrate, the clinical care provided to patients across providers and sites-of-care."

The regulatory definition promulgated by the US Department of Justice and the Federal Trade Commission (FTC) (US Department of Justice and the Federal Trade Commission 1996) in the "Statements of Antitrust Enforcement Policy in Health Care" states that clinical integration is "an active and ongoing program to evaluate and modify practice patterns by the network's physician participants and create a high degree of interdependence and cooperation among physicians to control costs and ensure quality."

The FTC's definition provides the framework for a collaborative care and contracting model that was intended to allow a framework for organizations to go beyond the popular "messenger model" adopted in the 1990s by many physician-hospital organizations (PHOs). Since 1996, a variety of healthcare organizations have followed the guidance provided in the FTC's statements and developed coordinated healthcare networks that allow for joint contracting among otherwise competing providers, in many cases between hospitals and both their employed and affiliated (independent) medical staff.

The Advisory Board (2012) defines *clinical integration* as "a network of physicians working (most often) in collaboration with a hospital [that] includes a program of initiatives to improve the quality and efficiency of patient care, developed and managed by physicians, and supported by a performance management infrastructure. Clinical integration provides a legal basis for collective negotiation by independent physicians for improved reimbursement on the basis of improved clinical outcomes and efficiency."

Advocate Health Care (2012) provides insight into its philosophy on clinical integration: "In our unique Clinical Integration Program, physicians work together to address the quality and costs associated with an entire episode of care—not just one visit. Physicians also work directly with patients to reduce the physical and financial effects of disease and illness by designing treatment plans that include medical intervention and lifestyle changes."

According to consulting firm BDC Advisors (Anderson, Wieland, and Spiegel 2011), "Clinical integration is a critical stage in a health system's transition to 'accountable care.'"

Despite the many definitions for clinical integration, a common theme emerges: quality improvement facilitated by physician engagement and leadership. The

Exhibit 9.1: Key Meaningful Clinical Integration Elements

Categories of Clinical Integration
Clinical Model Primary care physicians and specialists are in formal care management systems using concepts incorporated in Medicare Shared Savings ACOs and medical homes. Ultimate goal is clinical improvement in quality and providing the right care at the right time in the right place. May or may not have FTC approval.
Business Model A legal contracting entity that is able to bill, manage, track, and distribute payments from diverse payer contracts, including fee-for-service, value-based, and capitation. Ultimate goal is to develop business contracts that secure coverage for provider services. May or may not have FTC approval.
Federal Trade Commission (FTC) Definition
Clinical integration is a model of a physician–hospital contract that ◆ is based on development of a robust quality improvement program with real accountability among otherwise independent physicians, ◆ integrates and rewards physician members around a common commitment to quality measures based on scientific evidence, and ◆ has some form of FTC review.

remainder of this chapter is designed to provide a brief overview of a high-level approach to clinical integration, building the CIO.

Two categories of clinical integration exist—(1) legal/regulatory and (2) clinical/business—and they exist for two different reasons (see Exhibit 9.1). The legal and regulatory definition is significantly influenced by the more narrow FTC model requirements, which primarily relate to the organizational (CIO/ACO) goal of jointly contracting for the provision of services and avoiding violations of antitrust law. The second, broader clinical and business definition incorporates significant involvement of physicians, hospitals, and other healthcare providers using advanced clinical models that inherently drive greater value for clinical services provided while demonstrating higher levels of quality. The ability to deliver value-based clinical, business, and insurance models resides with effective execution of both aspects of clinical integration.

Advocate Health Care meets both definitions of a CIO. Lee B. Sacks, MD (2010), Advocate's chief medical officer, states that the following are critical success factors in clinical integration:

- Being physician driven
- Using the same metrics across all payers
- Minimizing additional administrative costs
- Providing additional funds to recognize extra work by physicians and staff
- Maintaining the infrastructure necessary to support improvement
- Practicing physician/hospital alignment

Note the common theme throughout these definitions and approaches: physician involvement and leadership to improve patient quality and clinical effectiveness.

WHAT A CIO PROVIDES

A CIO ultimately means that physicians, hospitals, and other providers must share accountability for patients as they move from one setting of care to another over the entire course of their care. The benefits for the patient include the elimination of duplicate clinical and administrative work, a common patient record that ensures that the status of the patient is tracked throughout the entire course of care with no continuity-of-care gaps, a reduced chance of errors, systematic support of best practices and evidence-based care, and full alignment of the goals of all providers.

And from a business perspective, a CIO is a good structure for holding a value-based contract—which falls somewhere between full economic integration that allows an entity to bear risk as an organization on the one end and accepting pure fee-for-service, which has little additional revenue stream incentives, on the other. A CIO, or an ACO, significantly expands the number and size of revenue streams available to an entity by allowing doctors and hospitals to hold value-based contracts that, in addition to providing substantially expanded revenue streams, do not require the rigor of economically integrated, capitated, or percent-of-premium contracts or relationships.

The many changes occurring over the next few years will be significant. To describe all of them in detail is beyond the scope of this book. However, to address the need for enhanced physician leadership, we provide the following historical background.

CHANGE IN HEALTHCARE: PAST, PRESENT, AND FUTURE

Dramatic changes are occurring in the healthcare system, and they started long before the Patient Protection and Affordable Care Act (ACA) was enacted. Costs are too high. Patients are crowding already overburdened provider organizations. Neither the government health system nor the private system has enough money. And several key healthcare professions are facing serious personnel shortages. Futurist Nate Kaufman (2012) predicts that "hospitals will become more accountable and exposed to increased penalties for care." These penalties will take the form of requiring more accountability metrics for the patient experience within the institution, provision of healthcare services in the CIO, and defined quality metrics identified by payers (e.g., CMS, private insurers).

Government intervention is nothing new, and neither is the feeling that efforts to control costs are akin to banging one's head—hard—against a brick wall.

- The Balanced Budget Act of 1997 established a sustainable growth rate for federal healthcare programs, but it now represents more than $300 billion in unfunded liabilities related to physician reimbursement rates.
- The Medicare Modernization Act of 2003 created the Part D prescription drug benefit and hastened the transition to more meaningful use of diagnosis-related groups.
- The Deficit Reduction Act of 2005 decreased reimbursement for office-based ancillary services as of 2007.
- The Tax Relief and Health Care Act of 2006 created Medicare medical home projects in eight states as of 2009.
- The ACA, passed in 2010, adds approximately 32 million Americans to insurance rolls through expanded Medicare and Medicaid programs and the creation of health insurance exchanges (HIEs)—meaning only about 23 million Americans will be without coverage, mostly undocumented workers and those who opt not to seek coverage.
- Effective October 1, 2012, hospitals can receive penalties from CMS for certain readmissions, poor performance on core measures of clinical care, and low patient satisfaction scores on the Medicare Hospital Consumer Assessment of Healthcare Providers and Systems (HCAHPS) survey.

All healthcare organizations face profound changes from legislation, regulations, guidelines, and judicial opinions and rulings.

Value Replaces Volume

CMS has defined *value-based purchasing* as any program that "links payment more directly to the quality of care provided." CMS adopted this approach as a "strategy that can help to transform the current payment system by rewarding providers for delivering high quality, efficient clinical care" (CMS 2007). Essentially, the objective of CMS and any other payer who desires to enter into value-based payments is to improve quality and efficiency of care. Some of the specific targets of these programs include the prevention of acute episodes in patients who have health conditions; prevention of bad outcomes during major acute episodes, such as infections, complications, and hospital readmissions; and reducing waste and inefficiency. A key change in the ACA is its emphasis on value-based reimbursement over the traditional fee-for-service methodology. The two systems are contrasted in the following box.

Fee-for-Service System

1. Hospital the primary setting for care
2. Rewards volume—more tests and procedures (more "heads in beds")
3. Features a less-than-optimal distinction of differences in quality of care, even with typical performance metrics
4. Contracting often done sporadically; multiple contracts; not all providers together in a single-signature contract arrangement
5. Spotlights inequities in access
6. Limits physician–patient face time for dealing with complex or challenging conditions
7. Discourages coordination of care over time and across the continuum of care
8. Undermines strong physician–patient relationships and team-based care

Value-Based Payment System

1. Physician office (or patient home) the primary setting for care
2. Rewards value and provides fewer services (fewer "heads in beds")
3. Positions CIOs to optimize quality requirements
4. Structures CIOs not just as a new version of a physician–hospital organization or a new contracting entity but with real "clinical glue" so that value-based payment stands up to FTC antitrust review
5. Encourages mobility of care: taking the right care to the right place as well as optimizing existing brick-and-mortar facilities
6. Pays for care management
7. Pays for evidence-based care; ties payments to measurable standards that are clear to both providers and consumers
8. Increases care delivery in a team-based model

CIOs PROVIDE THE STRUCTURE FOR CHANGE

While the terms *CIO* and *ACO* are often used interchangeably, they are different. ACOs generally involve the federal government (e.g., CMS/Medicare Shared Saving Programs) or a state-based payment sponsor (e.g., State of Massachusetts), while CIOs are more varied and flexible and participate with multiple private and public payers (e.g., Blue Shield of California, Aetna). CIOs may serve both as the beginning steps toward full integration (getting physicians on board with focus on quality improvement) and as end goals (having a fully functioning cohesive organization of all providers ready to accept all types of payment mechanisms). Do not let the various definitions get in the way of taking aggressive steps toward implementation of these value-based models.

Redding (2012) suggests that the main differences between CIOs and ACOs are as follows:

- CIOs tend to focus on developing a business case to substantiate premium payments from commercial payers via joint contracting.
- ACOs tend to focus on realizing incremental revenues through hybrid shared savings and pay-for-performance incentive programs.
- An ACO may or may not be a CIO. A successful CIO may or may not function as an ACO, but a successful ACO will have to be a CIO.

Note as well that there are differences between Medicare Shared Savings Program ACOs, which are tightly prescribed, and commercial ACOs, which offer more variety.

CIOs usually will

- be a legal entity, such as a limited liability company or a 501(c)(3), that can enter into all types of physician–hospital reimbursement contractual relationships, including fee-for-service, value-based payment, and capitation;
- have as a priority achieving "meaningful clinical integration" status by 2014—as reviewed by the FTC, the Department of Justice, and the Department of Health and Human Services—to participate in state-based health insurance exchanges; and
- support next-generation care models compatible with participation in or sponsorship of ACOs, CMS bundled payment programs, and patient-centered medical home initiatives.

> In my opinion, the true characteristic that makes clinical integration the "optimal" vehicle is its nonprescriptive nature. Unlike any other model, it is a business-case-based model that allows for flexibility, adaptability, and innovation.
> —*John Redding,*
> *2012*

Common Elements of Hospital or Health System CIOs

CIOs share the following elements:

- Physicians, both employed and independent (or in some cases, all employed), working together
- Physician practices integrated with hospital practices
- A multispecialty culture among all physician specialties
- Key independent ancillary services integrated into the mix
- An effective electronic health record (EHR) with strong data warehousing capabilities
- An evolving interface between the health system and payers that requires clinical integration

Legal Considerations

The meaningful clinical integration structure is further defined by the agreements between the hospital, its employed physicians, and the independent physicians with whom it contracts. The integrated providers negotiate jointly with payers for base reimbursement, shared savings, and performance incentives. (The information provided in this chapter is for informational purposes only and not for the purpose of providing legal advice. You should contact an attorney to obtain advice about any particular issue or problem.) These arrangements bring up several important legal considerations.

Market power concentration. Organizations are faced with the paradox that, while the government is encouraging integration, it is also challenging arrangements that may reduce competition. Mergers that materially reduce competition may be subject to challenge. No clear benchmarks exist, but if the CIO gains too much market share, aggrieved parties (e.g., competitors, purchasers of services) may find a receptive audience with the FTC. That assessment will be based on the definition of the relevant market, which is the product of both geography and competitive alternatives.

Fraud and abuse issues. CIOs must be aware of the Anti-Kickback Statute (42 USC Section 1320a-7b(b)) , the Stark law and regulations, and their implications. Basically, CIOs cannot pay for referrals. They must also have commercially reasonable, fair-market-value contractual arrangements that do not compensate the service provider on the basis of volume or for the value of referrals.

Licensing and regulatory issues. Although the laws differ from state to state, corporate practice of medicine prohibitions generally forbid business corporations from practicing medicine and, in some states, do not allow a physician to be employed by a business corporation to provide professional medical services. Bans on fee splitting also prohibit physicians from sharing professional fees with lay entities.

Operational Considerations

The CIO's organizational parameters include the following:

- **Clinical scope:** Encompasses the full continuum of care, including both inpatient and outpatient settings
- **Membership:** Targets physicians whose participation has the potential to maximize quality and efficient resource utilization
- **Performance improvement:** Designed to improve quality and reduce costs through adherence to protocols that are supported by comprehensive data collection and reporting
- **A robust EHR system**
- **Capital requirements:** Significant investment to develop and deploy a technology infrastructure—both clinical and financial—to support improved care delivery. Capital requirements vary widely depending on whether a CIO or ACO wishes to build, buy, or partner infrastructure and work process functionality.

Physician to Physician

Don't let the introduction of clinical integration get too complicated. Physicians will understand its underpinnings and rationale. Be sure you keep the steps simple and bite sized. Make sure the physicians can see the two or three clear end-point objectives for creating the CIO right from the start.
—Jacque Sokolov, MD

The structure of a CIO often involves tiered networks with different financial elements for each. Each tier represents movement along the clinical integration spectrum. As integration increases, on the way from fee-for-service at one extreme to value-based payment at the other, so does financial risk. And that is how the regulators—who want providers to carry more financial risk for their actions—seem to want it. The four tiers are as follows:

- Tier 1: The baseline large network, must be compliant with FTC guidelines and be compatible with a meaningful clinical integration infrastructure
- Tier 2: Smaller than Tier 1 and capable of managing more advanced clinical integration requirements, including PCP care management payments, Medicare Shared Savings Program, quality performance targets, and more
- Tier 3: Smaller than Tier 2 and capable of receiving global payments for initiatives, including pay-for-performance
- Tier 4: Smaller than Tier 3 and capable of accepting global payments with steep financial risk for the providers involved

For example, a commercial health plan's Tier 1 network could be configured as an employee health plan governed by the Employee Retirement Income Security Act (ERISA). Its Tier 2 and Tier 3 networks could serve as the basis for an ACO (Exhibit 9.2) or an administrative services-only plan; similarly, they could be configured as an ERISA-covered employee benefit plan and as a non-HIE-based value-based purchasing plan. Separately, the Tier 3 network could service a state-based HIE plan. The Tier 4 network could be configured for a Medicare Advantage plan.

CONCLUSION

Healthcare executives must face the fact that their environment is changing dramatically, and the old days of unfettered fee-for-service are never coming back. Seemingly every change in the healthcare industry is pushing provider organizations—hospitals, physicians, and other providers alike—into alliances and collaborative efforts they would never have thought necessary as recently as a decade ago. The answer is out there, though. It is called a clinically integrated organization, and all the pieces are already in place. Now leaders in healthcare must stitch the pieces together in a way that provides value to payers and patients. As CIOs and ACOs become common practice, healthcare organizations will be confronted with the need to use physicians to a greater degree, use EHR and data warehousing to better track quality of care and outcomes, deploy patient-centered medical homes, and monitor the performance of physicians, providers, and hospitals. The clarion call is for enhanced physician involvement and leadership is clearly here to maximize the value of the CIO.

Exhibit 9.2: Potential ACO Model

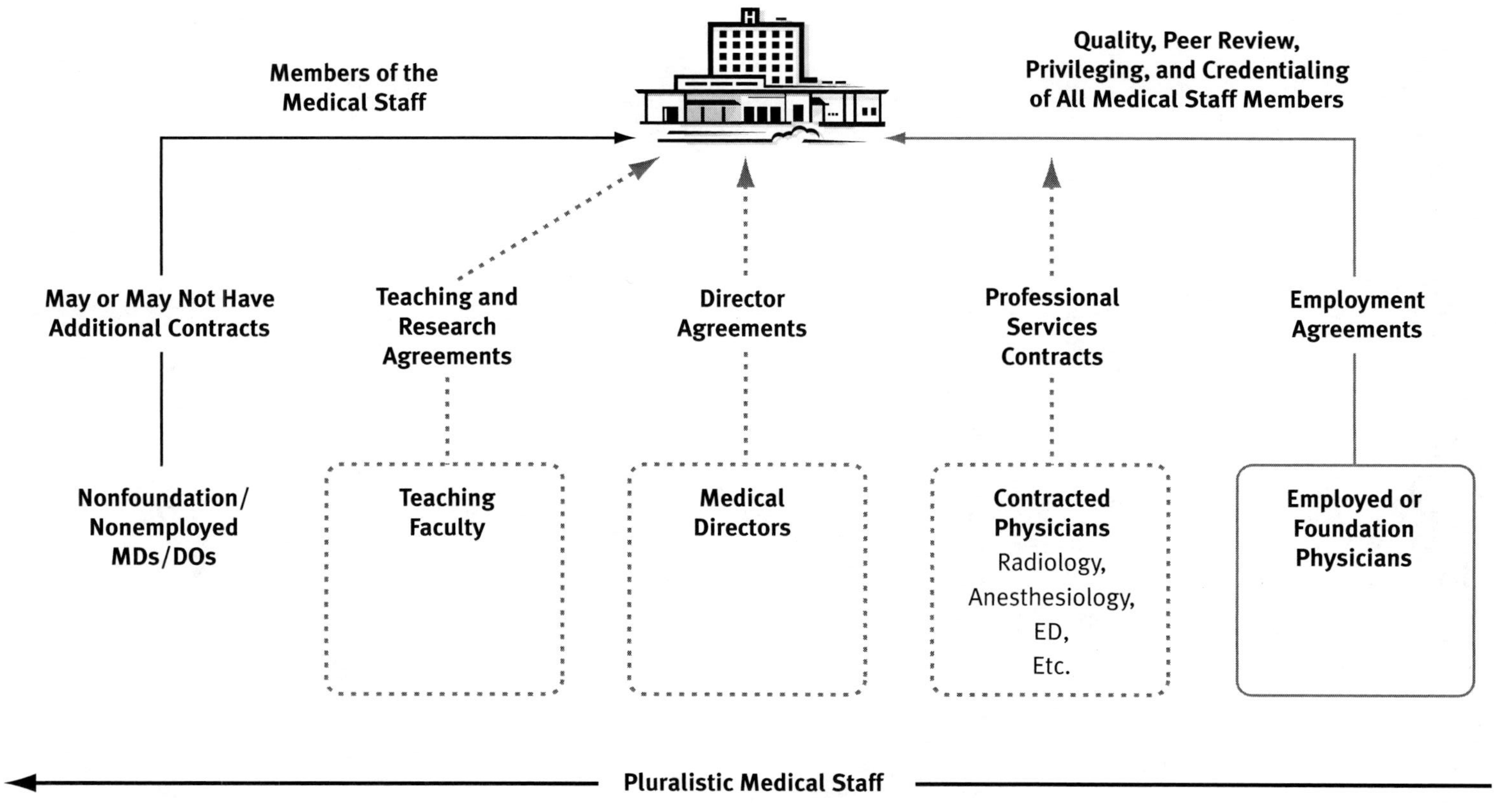

Quality, Peer Review, Privileging, and Credentialing of All Medical Staff Members

Members of the Medical Staff

May or May Not Have Additional Contracts

Employment Agreements — Employed or Foundation Physicians

Professional Services Contracts — Contracted Physicians
Radiology, Anesthesiology, ED, Etc.

Director Agreements — Medical Directors

Teaching and Research Agreements — Teaching Faculty

Nonfoundation / Nonemployed MDs / DOs

Pluralistic Medical Staff

Thoughts for Consideration

Where would your organization fall on a sliding scale from "operating in the past" to "fully embracing the future"?

What economic factors are driving your organization to clinical integration?

What factors in your specific market are pushing you in that direction?

Does your organization have—or can it find in the market—the expertise necessary to form close relationships with physicians across broad clinical categories of care?

Does your organization fully understand how CIOs are formed and operated? Do your physicians have a good grasp of the fundamentals?

SUGGESTED READING

Bohn, J. M. 2011. *Your Next Steps in Healthcare Transformation*. Louisville, KY: Touchcast Press.

de Marco, W. J. 2011. *Performance-Based Medicine: Creating the High-Performance Network to Optimize Managed Care Relationships.* London: Productivity Press.

Flareau, B., J. M. Bohn, and C. Konschak. 2011. *Accountable Care Organizations: A Roadmap for Success: Guidance on First Steps*. Virginia Beach, VA: Convurgent Publishing LLC.

Flareau, B., K. Yale, C. Konschak, and J. M. Bohn. 2011. *Clinical Integration: A Roadmap to Accountable Care.* 2nd ed. Virginia Beach, VA: Convurgent Publishing.

CHAPTER 10

Building a Clinically Integrated Organization: A How-To Guide

Hospital Executive A: We've officially taken the plunge. We've woken up and smelled the proverbial coffee, and now we're moving toward clinical integration.

Hospital Executive B: Fabulous. We're also sitting on Go, ready to start our own integration efforts, but we're looking for a role model of sorts. How is your effort going?

Hospital Executive A: We started with our physicians, of course. It just makes sense to build a physician-focused entity around physicians, as they're both the most challenging element of an integration effort and, at the same time, its very foundation.

Hospital Executive B: Amen to that. I suppose putting a strong administrative structure in place comes next, right?

Hospital Executive A: Indeed. We've done that, too. Now we're looking at the final phase, actually aligning our clinical products and services. Wish us luck!

Nothing about clinical integration is really new or fundamentally difficult. But it is a process that takes focus, effort, and extreme tact. The phases of clinical integration are what you would expect: Assemble your frontline providers and establish them in important leadership positions; put an overall administrative infrastructure in place; and then integrate your clinical products and services. Do not be intimidated—each step in the process is achievable. Just be aware that new structures of governance, management, and operations will need to be created, and old ones will need to be modified or discarded.

In Chapter 9, we looked at the environmental underpinnings of the healthcare industry's move to clinical integration and at what makes up a clinically integrated organization (CIO). In this chapter, we provide a brief overview of how to construct a CIO. Building a CIO generally occurs in three phases and with four discrete projects (see Exhibit 10.1).

A physician organization project is part of the first phase, which gives physicians insight into how the operating entity would be structured and, most important, helps physicians see the need for combining forces and collaborating with one another and the sponsoring organization (usually a hospital or health system). A CIO administrative project makes up the second phase. The third phase, the pure clinical integration of previously less-connected product lines and services, includes a medical staff collaboration project and a clinical model (we call this the "model of the future" project because it represents the ultimate end goal structure).

PHASE ONE

The first phase of CIO development includes numerous levels at which hospitals and physicians can collaborate (see "Levels of Clinical Integration"); given the changes occurring in healthcare, market drivers and reimbursement shifts will push the delivery system toward greater clinical integration. Readers will note the use of the word *collaborate* rather than *integrate*. The authors contend that past efforts to integrate often suggested that physicians lost their identity as they became integrated and were converted into cogs in the corporate healthcare enterprise. This situation created much of the distrust and contentiousness we have seen over the past several years. In the world of clinical integration, this is not the case; in fact, physicians lead the process.

Levels of Clinical Integration

1. Contractual ties
2. Payer contracting
3. Key practice support
4. Joint ventures and comanagement models
5. Full clinical integration
6. Physician employment
7. CIO

Exhibit 10.1: Phases of Building a CIO

Phase One	**Physician Organization Project: The Intro**
	Getting physicians ready for the new operating entity, helping them see the changes ahead, and engaging them in supporting the development of the ultimate clinical integration model ♦ Education ♦ Engagement ♦ Deciding whether to develop a formal physician organization ♦ Attention to the aligned and nonaligned physician dynamic
Phase Two	**CIO Administration Project: The Form**
	Transforming health systems into value-based CIOs, getting the legal and administrative i's dotted and the t's crossed, and developing the infrastructure that will allow the physicians to participate ♦ Legal structure ♦ Organization ♦ Governance ♦ Committee structure ♦ Care delivery transformation ♦ Infrastructure development ♦ Budgeting and financial modeling
Phase Three	**Medical Staff Collaboration Project: The Substance**
	Getting the physicians actively involved in the formal process, signing them up as participants in the corporate structure, and getting their buy-in to participate in quality and cost data sharing ♦ Education ♦ Engagement ♦ Discussions around the proper structure for collaboration ♦ Delegated functionality
	Clinical Model: The Model of the Future
	Designing and implementing the final organizational structure and using data to enhance quality and efficiency, picking up the first contracts, and getting the feet wet with quality and financial performance ♦ Provider compensation ♦ Clinical transformation ♦ Technology enablement ♦ Contract negotiation ♦ Mobility of care elements in nontraditional settings

In the most basic level of integration, collaboration means *contractual ties* only—say, where physicians serve as medical directors and provide clinical and quality guidance in patient areas. In general, specialists are more involved at this level than are primary care physicians (PCPs). The contractual ties are specific to a single physician or group for designated services. The strategic value of the contractual ties is low, as is the level of complexity and risk. Fee-for-service reimbursement dominates.

In the next level of integration, providers join together for *payer contracting*. This strategy is a move that is designed to increase providers' negotiating strength but has become increasingly ineffective. These types of collaborative relationships —which often take the form of a physician–hospital organization (PHO)—generally involve a mix of PCPs and specialists. The level of complexity and risk from this model increases proportionally as the market share of physician and hospital services increases within a discrete geographic area. Fee-for-service reimbursement continues to dominate.

The third level of integration involves *key practice support* ties, including management services organizations, loans, and recruiting support designed to assist independent physicians and group practices. PCPs tend to be better represented in such ties than specialists. The level of complexity and risk continues to focus on market share contracting concentration and "fair market value" for any services provided in this integration model. The strategic value of these relationships and services remains of value to the mutual parties (physicians and hospitals). Fee-for-service reimbursement still dominates.

The fourth level of integration involves *joint ventures* or *comanagement models*, such as imaging centers or ambulatory surgery centers, with specialists. Joint ventures are economic partnerships in which the assets or services are jointly owned by the physicians and the hospital. The level of complexity and risk is noticeably higher than for the other types of collaboration, and the strategic value is quite a bit higher. A comanagement model is essentially an arrangement in which hospitals enter into management agreements that have physicians manage hospital service lines. A comanagement model provides incentives for physicians in the development, management, and improvement of quality and efficiency and also in making the service line more competitive in the market. Fee-for-service reimbursement dominates, but glimmers of value-based reimbursement may be seen in especially sophisticated specialty comanagement arrangements.

The final level for clinical integration is a full-fledged CIO (see "Accountable Care and Clinical Integration"). A CIO is a physician–hospital alignment entity involving specialists and PCPs that enables clinical integration needed for value-based contracting and for passing Federal Trade Commission (FTC) review. The level of complexity and risk is much higher than it is for the other levels of integration, and the strategic value is higher as well.

At the high end of the integration scale is *physician employment*—by the hospital, a larger physician group, or a related organization, such as a payer—and its variations; an even mix of specialists and PCPs is usually involved. The level of complexity and risk of such ties is as high as it gets, as is the strategic value of the ties.

Accountable Care and Clinical Integration

Where do accountable care organizations (ACOs) fall on the integration scale? CIOs and ACOs both have high levels of complexity and risk and require an aligned physician group. The predominant difference is that an ACO is defined by the Centers for Medicare & Medicaid Services (CMS) as a Medicare Shared Savings organization with specific integration waivers allowing physicians and hospitals certain relationships that would not normally be afforded non-ACO participants. CIOs are ACOs that can accept value-based payment from multiple payers and do not have the CMS ACO waiver protection. The strategic value for ACOs and CIOs is their ability to function in a value-based reimbursement structure. They are organizations with a payment and care delivery model that links reimbursements to quality and reduced cost of care. A CIO or ACO may use capitation, fee-for-service, or some type of shared savings model of payment for the services, depending on the payer.

Physician Leadership and Engagement at Multiple Levels

A CIO requires physician leadership in multiple areas:

- **Governance.** Physician leadership is required at the board of managers or board of directors level. Physicians should chair and play lead roles in subcommittees, such as the quality committee.
- **Management.** A strong CEO or president (physician or nonphysician) is key to accelerating and managing physician engagement at all levels. Although some would disagree, the authors believe that physicians must be at the head.
- **Operations.** The clinical and financial performance of medical groups, independent practice associations, and provider networks must be driven by physi-

cians who clearly understand clinical and financial endpoint expectations. Performance evaluations of practicing clinicians should be done by physicians.

- **Patient population.** CIOs and ACOs have specific physician leadership needs related to developing sophisticated care models for complex senior and special-needs populations.
- **Value-based purchasing requirements.** Physician leadership is required to assess the ability to implement value-based purchasing exchange products.

One Example of a CIO

One southwestern health network CIO with four owners (a seven-hospital system, a hospital-sponsored medical group, a dedicated physician network, and an independent practice association) operates as a taxable not-for-profit entity that integrates hospital services and the multiple types of physician practices. (A taxable not-for-profit engages in some business activities that are unrelated to its nonprofit status, thus it pays taxes on that income.) A hospital-sponsored medical group represents employed physicians working together and includes about 100 PCPs and about 900 specialists. Alongside the employed physician group, the CIO physician network consisting of independent physicians and the IPA make up the overall CIO physician network. As the organization moves toward meaningful clinical integration, its evolving interface with payers, including the mix of fee-for-service and value-based reimbursement, reinforces increasing clinical integration.

PHASE TWO

In the second phase of CIO development, health systems transforming into value-based CIOs must focus on essential components. The project will require multiple workgroups, task forces, and a great deal of structured interface with physician leadership. The project should address the following issues:

- **Organizational or governance structure.** Create a "one enterprise" culture for shared accountability, risks, and rewards.
- **Organizational infrastructure.** Focus on administrative services, budgeting and financial modeling, a clinical model, an operational model, and information technology needs.

- **Network development.** Develop and mature the CIO network to align across the health plan and CMS product continuum to enable maximum health system flexibility and options.
- **Care delivery transformation.** The clinical models will change, with an increased emphasis on implementation of evidence-based practices, patient engagement, seamless care transitions, and capacity optimization.
- **Payer contract restructuring.** In the short term, restructuring means adding sufficient size and scope to the delivery system to enhance its attractiveness to payers. In the intermediate term, it means collaborating with government, private payers, and employers to reward value and build accountability for managing healthcare quality and costs. In the long term, it means being accountable for the entire health of a defined population (a stage few organizations will have the size to accomplish).

Another example of a CIO joint venture structure could merge the physician members, organized under a physician limited liability company (LLC) with up to 50 percent ownership, and the hospital or health system, likely a 501(c)(3) or LLC with 50 to 100 percent ownership, into an integrated entity, either a CIO or an ACO, that is wholly owned by the health system or a joint venture with the physicians. This entity provides management services, and it contracts with payers and CMS for care management fees, physician value-based performance, and, ultimately, for "single signature" agreements (agreements that bind both hospitals and providers to a common contract with a payer).

Such CIOs share the savings they achieve through clinical integration and better-focused care management. A percentage goes to specialist groups, and a percentage goes to primary care groups in the form of per-member-per-month fees. The rest of the savings goes to the hospital. The amount that is split, the CIO's value-based reimbursement, is based on mutual shared savings and meeting quality metrics. Some CIOs have dozens of value-based purchasing metrics; some commercial-based products are pushing toward more than 100 quality metrics. Already, the Medicaid program is moving to value-based purchasing metrics.

Costs of Developing a CIO

The costs of developing a CIO occur in multiple categories:

- Physician alignment strategies may entail hospital-sponsored medical group (also called an employed physician network) development (Exhibit 10.2),

Exhibit 10.2: Hospital-Sponsored Medical Group Structural Options

Three Basic Structures	
Model A: Embedded Medical Group	A hospital-sponsored medical group is a virtual stand-alone medical group with an advisory board, physician executive, and chief administrative officer, but embedded in a health system structure.
Model B: Separate Medical Group	Not a virtual stand-alone medical group, it is structured as a separate 501(c)(3) or LLC legal entity sponsored by a stand-alone health system.
Model C: Medical Foundation Model (Most commonly found in states subject to the corporate practice of medicine laws)	The medical group is structured as a separate for-profit entity, with a contract to provide clinical services for a discrete period. The foundation established by the health system houses all the assets and personnel of previously autonomous medical groups.

*Note: Many other variations exist (including legacy models, foundation-owned medical groups, for-profit medical groups, exclusive professional services models, and more), but these three models are the most common.

comanagement specialty entities, service line bundled payments, medical home development, or a combination of all four. The total costs vary according to the number and type of alignment methods but will include legal, consulting, and administrative costs as well as ongoing operational costs.

♦ Organizational development includes planning, legal and other related services, and its regulatory compliance. Costs go to legal and consulting support.

♦ Payer contracting and network development requires staffing support. Costs go to salaries and management fees.

♦ Care management includes development of protocols, benchmarks, and standards. Costs go to licensing, software, and personnel.

♦ Informatics include information technology and health insurance exchange–necessitated infrastructure. Costs go to hardware, software, and licensing.

♦ Health plan services and third-party administration (TPA) includes core health plan and administration services, such as claims management and financial tracking. Costs are paid by the payer or other TPA partner.

- Physician education and training (e.g., for managing the medical staff interface) includes development and transformation of a clinical model and performance metrics. Costs go to compensation for modeling, development, and other support.

PHASE THREE

The final phase of CIO development includes the physician collaboration project and establishing the clinical model. The fact that three of the four discrete projects embedded in the three phases are physician-centric explains why physician leadership is so essential to meaningful clinical integration—and why physician organization-centric decisions are necessary.

In gaining physician engagement, remember the following:

- Physician organization-centric decisions are key. Use a "boots on the ground" approach that involves physicians at every level of the organization. This is not the time for top-down mandates; physicians need to be meaningfully involved in all meetings and moments of decision.
- Physician-centric decisions are vital. The decisions that will be made will have significant impact on how physicians practice and take care of their patients. The decisions can cause administrative and time burdens, and physicians must be at the strategy and decision-making table.
- Moving to a CIO clinical model is a transformative and evolutionary process. The model involves the right care at the right place at the right time, and emphasizes care mobility and patient satisfaction. Organizations will not reach this endpoint in a few months; it likely will take two to three years of concerted efforts.

Keep in mind one central facet of physicians: They generally do *not* want someone to advocate for them, even when that other person is a physician; physicians want to advocate for themselves.

CIOs start with a physician organization focus and often with physician organization functions. In some cases, a physician umbrella organization (PUO) serves as the best organizing vehicle to facilitate and coordinate physician equity and governance participation in the CIO. The PUO sits between the physician organization's board and the independent, contracted, and employed physicians who serve the CIO's patients.

Functions of the PUO include

- serving as a vehicle for physician capital contributions and investment in the CIO;
- selecting physician representatives for the CIO board;
- determining physicians' positions on key policy issues and communicating those positions to the CIO physician board members;
- expediting two-way communication between the CIO board and physicians;
- educating physicians regarding the advantages of participating in the PUO and the CIO; and
- recruiting physicians to participate in the PUO and the CIO.

In many cases, the other role of the PUO is to support the organization's clinical governance council to hold membership accountable for clinical performance, ensuring membership standards are upheld (particularly in credentialing) and that quality targets are met.

Limitations of the Traditional Medical Staff Model

Many readers have experienced the types of medical staff meetings during which it is difficult to keep order, stay focused on an agenda, and avoid discussions turning into gripe sessions. Some of those meetings no doubt erupted into shouting matches and at times ended with great divisions. As health systems move toward tighter clinical integration, they need to fine-tune and expand the existing physician governance and decision-making structure to minimize the effects of these types of meetings. The agenda must be more focused on how to solidify a tightly integrated delivery system across the care continuum emphasizing quality and efficiency. Moreover, most medical staff structures today are not designed to handle the issues of physician employment and CIOs. Current structures generally include a hospital board delegating responsibility for the medical staff to a medical executive committee, which then interacts with medical staff departments, while the hospital CEO is left somewhere outside that chain of authority. Further compounding the problem is the existence of increasing numbers of employed physicians who may or may not fall under the oversight of the medical staff. The core problem is that hospital boards and management have limited authority to drive change to enable greater clinical quality, operational efficiency, and effectiveness.

While many options exist, we feel that a better CIO–medical staff governance collaboration model starts with the end in mind and features a system board with authority over the quality committee and the clinical integration committee (CIC).

CIC subcommittees include system credentialing, system quality, and system peer review. The quality committee and CIC interface with executive leadership and the CEO, and both work well with the system board. Feeding into the various quality and clinical integration committees are a physicians council (representing the medical executive committees and the system hospitals) and various advisory boards (representing the other elements of the system, including health plans, other physicians, and specialty products and services).

The Importance of Care Coordination

A patient-centered medical home (PCMH) is likely to be one of the key component parts of a CIO. It functions as the care coordination model for the CIO. Although several definitions exist, the best defines a PCMH as a system rooted in primary care that uses a primary care physician to manage patient care and services. It requires a care team that may involve the use of physician extenders such as nurse practitioners, mechanisms to get patients actively involved in their care, enhanced patient access, use of a disease registry, and coordination of care across the continuum (see Exhibit 10.3). The American Academy of Family Physicians (2012) defines a PCMH as "an ongoing, active partnership with a personal primary care physician who leads a team of professionals dedicated to providing proactive, preventive and chronic care management through all stages of life." The term originated in 1967 when the American Academy of Pediatrics suggested the concept to refer to pediatric patients' medical records being archived in a central location.

How does the CIO PCMH work in practice?

Care coordination is central to any clinical integration effort. Patients are stratified according to a variety of data sources, including claims, prescriptions, labs, referrals, medical records, emergency room admissions, and health reimbursement accounts. Health status is divided into low-risk patients who require acute episodic care but mostly routine health maintenance; medium-risk patients, for whom a diagnosis may be unknown but whose chronic disease is stable; and high-risk patients, whose chronic disease is unstable or changing and who have been recently hospitalized.

Care coordination and the success of clinical integration is ultimately determined and sustained by several components (see Exhibit 10.4). The exhibit shows how the various components work together to enhance quality.

Care coordination varies by health status. In all cases, it involves personal physicians, care coordinators, and allied health professionals. For low-risk patients, episodic outreach is adequate. For medium-risk patients, mostly episodic outreach suffices, supplemented with occasional monthly interventions. High-risk patients

Exhibit 10.3: Patient-Centered Medical Home

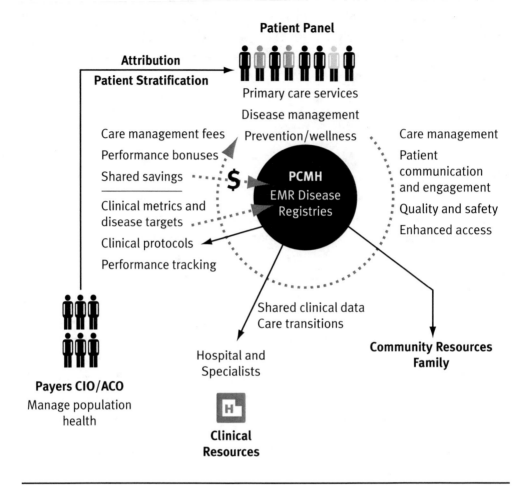

often require weekly or monthly interventions. Care coordination must provide both clinical management (including a sharp focus on patient outcomes and the clinical pathways that get them there) and resource management (including predictive modeling-based provider cost analyses and pay-for-performance benchmarks).

Legal Considerations

Many of the concepts introduced here and in Chapter 9 have multifaceted legal complexities. Readers should always consult competent legal counsel that has expertise in antitrust law and other laws.

We also present the material here and in Chapter 9 with the major focus of a hospital or heath system creating the CIO. We do so because the majority of CIOs

Exhibit 10.4: Key Components of Care Management Model

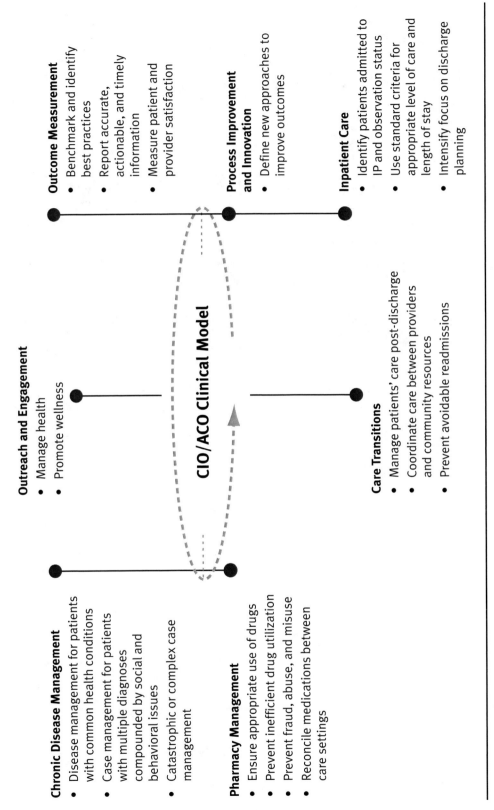

Outreach and Engagement
- Manage health
- Promote wellness

Outcome Measurement
- Benchmark and identify best practices
- Report accurate, actionable, and timely information
- Measure patient and provider satisfaction

Process Improvement and Innovation
- Define new approaches to improve outcomes

Inpatient Care
- Identify patients admitted to IP and observation status
- Use standard criteria for appropriate level of care and length of stay
- Intensify focus on discharge planning

CIO/ACO Clinical Model

Chronic Disease Management
- Disease management for patients with common health conditions
- Case management for patients with multiple diagnoses compounded by social and behavioral issues
- Catastrophic or complex case management

Pharmacy Management
- Ensure appropriate use of drugs
- Prevent inefficient drug utilization
- Prevent fraud, abuse, and misuse
- Reconcile medications between care settings

Care Transitions
- Manage patients' care post-discharge
- Coordinate care between providers and community resources
- Prevent avoidable readmissions

will likely emanate from hospitals or health systems. But recognize that CIOs can be formed without these organizations; IPAs or physician group practices may also do so. Moreover, recognize also that forms of CIOs may vary from the model described in these two chapters.

CONCLUSION

The steps to clinical integration really just make sense. Organizations can start by educating all levels of physicians about what the future holds and forming closer ties to physicians, whatever the contractual means. Then an administrative level is built on top, and efforts are made to be certain that clinical products and services complement, rather than compete with, each other. Although the execution may be difficult, the structure is simple, and physician leaders must be heavily involved in every activity.

Thoughts for Consideration

Which level of integration is your organization ready for? Are you still tying physicians in contractually? Have you moved to a physician–hospital organization for payer negotiations?

How would a PUO assist in your integration efforts?

Is a specialized CIO an option for your organization? For which clinical area or areas?

Should your organization form or participate in an ACO?

Do you have specific, discrete leadership opportunities for physicians at the governance, management, and operations levels? What are they?

SUGGESTED READING

Bader, B. S. 2009. "Clinically Integrated Physician-Hospital Organizations." *Great Boards.* Accessed September 25, 2012. www.greatboards.org/newsletter/2009/ Great-Boards-Winter-2009-reprint-Clinically-Integrated-PHOs.pdf.

Banghart, S. F. 2010. "Clinical Integration: Responding to Marketplace Realities and Changing Reimbursement Opportunities." Published March 1. *Ungaretti and Harris.* www.uhlaw.com/clinical-integration-responding-to-marketplace-realities-and-changing-reimbursement-opportunities-03-01-2010/.

Crosson, F. J., and L. A. Tollen. 2010. *Partners in Health: How Physicians and Hospitals Can Be Accountable Together.* Hoboken, NJ: Jossey-Bass.

Federal Trade Commission. 2008. "Clinical Integration in Health Care: A Check-Up." Federal Trade Commission Workshop on Health Care Clinical Integration, May 29. www.ftc.gov/bc/healthcare/checkup/index.shtm.

Marren, J. P. 2008. "Clinical Integration in Health Care: A Check-Up." *Federal Trade Commission.* Accessed November 4, 2012. www.ftc.gov/bc/healthcare/checkup/pdf/Marren%20Presentation%20-%20Clinical%20Integration%20Workshop.pdf.

Pizzo, J. J., and M. E. Grube. 2011. "Getting to There from Here: Evolving to ACOs Through Clinical Integration Programs." *Kaufman, Hall & Associates.* Accessed September 25, 2012. www.advocatehealth.com/documents/app/ci_to_aco.pdf.

Porter, M. E., and E. O. Teisberg. 2006. *Redefining Health Care: Creating Value-Based Competition on Results.* Boston: Harvard Business Review Press.

Redding, J. 2012. "4 Pitfalls to Clinical Integration." *Healthcare Financial Management Association.* Published November 1. http://www.hfma.org/Publications/hfm-Magazine/Archives/2012/November/4-Pitfalls-to-Clinical-Integration/.

Singer, T. 2008. "FTC Guidance on Clinical Integration: Comparison of Recent Advisory Opinions." *Federal Trade Commission.* Published May 29. www.ftc.gov/bc/healthcare/checkup/pdf/Marren%20Presentation%20-%20Clinical%20Integration%20Workshop.pdf.

Starling, K. G. 2011. "Antitrust Agencies Adopt Policy Statement on Medicare Accountable Care Organizations." *DLA Piper.* October 26. www.dlapiper.com/global/publications/Detail.aspx?pub=6466&RSS=true.

CHAPTER 11

The Enterprise Quality Plan: Structure, Function, and Physician Leadership Opportunities

Hospital Executive A: We've made a commitment to clinical integration, and that means we're more focused on quality than ever. We know that means relying on our affiliated physicians more than ever, but we could use a roadmap.

Hospital Executive B: I've got just what you need. An institution I'm familiar with in the Southwest has adopted a quality plan at the enterprise level. You'd be amazed at the opportunities for physician leadership it presents.

Hospital Executive A: Now, we don't want to hear about doctors taking over narrowly focused clinical departments, such as radiology or emergency medicine. We've been doing that for years.

Hospital Executive B: No, the institution I'm referring to has done much more than that. It has created leadership and management opportunities for physicians at the governance, management, and operations levels. There's really no part of the systemwide focus on quality that doesn't have at least one physician touch point.

Hospital Executive A: Tell me more!

The enterprise quality plan is both tactical and operational; it is a benchmark used for management and operational group performance that is reported annually to the board. The enterprise quality plan touches all the different pieces of the organization: the hospital, outpatient services, the employed medical group, and peer review and credentialing. It is a discrete plan, a

(continued)

---

management tool, and an operations tool that involves a significant number of physicians and nonphysicians, but it remains different from the structures of physician leadership that occur in governance, although it does have some crossover in its actual execution. The enterprise quality plan also carries multiple opportunities for physician leadership. Ideally, a physician serves on the board of directors, the chair of the board quality committee is a physician, and management-level physicians—such as the chief quality officer and chief medical officer—touch the quality plan. The physician–hospital organization piece involves the top physicians and the top nonphysicians working together and, ultimately, the plan all goes up to the board quality committee, which should have additional physician input.

The physician leadership rubber meets the clinically integrated quality management road at the enterprise quality plan. This expansive plan affects every aspect of a healthcare organization's governance, management, and operations—indeed, it affects just about every aspect of the enterprise in general—and it includes multiple options for physician leadership. The most productive way to look at clinical and quality initiatives in governance, management, and operations is to look at a case study that shows the structure, function, and deliverables of such a plan. This chapter looks at Phoenix Children's Hospital's (PCH) enterprise quality plan and its many physician leadership touch points.

DEVELOPING THE ENTERPRISE QUALITY PLAN

The enterprise quality plan at PCH consists of three components: quality and safety infrastructure and process, information technology infrastructure, and quality and safety measurement. Each of these has its own specific implementation steps, and each of those steps involves physician input (see "Clinical Expert Leadership Requirements") and continuing involvement.

Quality and Safety Infrastructure and Process

PCH included the following steps in its enterprise quality plan to create its quality and safety infrastructure:

1. Develop a core team dedicated to advancement of Lean principles for the organization. This step will include healthcare engineers who specialize in

streamlining processes and systems. Physician input is critical to ensure that process streamlining does not limit adequate care.

2. Regarding leadership, evaluate and make recommendations on the expected benefits of creating a vice president of quality or chief quality officer position. Physicians are in the best position to weigh the merits of each.

3. Assess and implement a physician practice management incentive compensation model using identified quality measures. Physician input here is, obviously, critical.

4. Assess and recommend potential roles of patients and families in initiatives that enhance patient care quality, service, and safety. As the coordinators of that care, physicians must provide input.

Clinical Expert Leadership Requirements

Of 12 specific steps in PCH's enterprise quality plan, the accountable executive for six (Steps 3, 5, 7, 9, 10, and 12) must be a physician. Four more (Steps 1, 2, 4, and 6) must be led by clinical experts, too—for example, the chief nursing officer (CNO) or the chief medical informatics officer (CMIO).

Quality and Safety Infrastructure and Process
- Senior vice president for clinical operations (a physician position)
- Chief medical officer (a physician position)
- Senior vice president representing the PCH Medical Group (a physician position)
- Vice president for human resources and chief nursing officer

Information Technology Infrastructure
- Chief medical informatics officer (not necessarily a physician, but a physician would better know what kind of data are needed)
- Chief information officer

Quality and Safety Measurement
- Chief medical officer
- Chief executive officer
- Chief financial officer
- The members of this effort—a wide variety of business and clinical leaders—all work collaboratively.

Information Technology Infrastructure

PCH recognized the importance of information management by adding these steps to its enterprise quality plan:

5. Assess and evaluate data analytics and reporting functionality to support quality initiatives. Only physicians can fully assess whether that functionality will actually accomplish what it should in supporting the enterprise quality plan.
6. Hire a dedicated IT analyst or analysts to meet electronic data needs for quality initiatives. Physicians should have input into all key hires for a quality program (and in some organizations, a physician CMIO will lead this area).
7. Implement comprehensive dose-range checking to improve medication safety. Physicians must, of course, have input into all specific clinical care-related quality programs.
8. Convert from manual to fully electronic data gathering, where available, to support quality improvement initiatives. Because they're most affected by such a conversion, physicians must have input into it.

Quality and Safety Measurement

Quality programs do not work in the long term if you cannot measure their success, so PCH added these steps to its quality enterprise plan:

9. Implement a transparency committee based on scope, charter, and membership specs approved by physicians.
10. Develop a targeted portfolio of regularly updated quality measures based on institutional priorities, for posting on the PCH intranet. Physicians should help in determining those priorities and in how the quality measures should be updated.
11. Identify and define measurement and monitoring methodologies for clinical outcomes and for indicators in the PCH "Strive for Zero" program to eliminate medical errors. As clinical experts, physician input into any and all outcomes measurement projects is essential.
12. Establish clinical and financial metrics relevant to value-based initiatives. Physician input into the clinical side of the equation is especially critical; otherwise, there may be too much emphasis on the financial side.

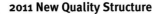

2011 New Quality Structure

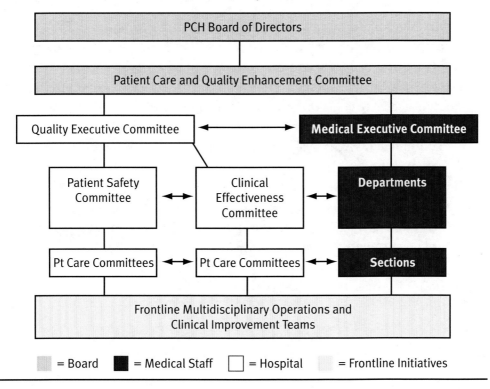

Physician involvement—representing significant *physician* management opportunities—is required in every step of this plan. PCH has realized substantial benefit in getting more physicians engaged.

Creating New Governance Leadership Opportunities

The enterprise quality plan at PCH called for forming three new committees as part of the restructuring of the quality-related committees of the hospital and medical staff: the quality executive committee (QEC), the patient safety committee, and the clinical effectiveness committee. As part of the restructuring, the hospital's existing transparency committee was combined with the QEC because of overlapping agendas and almost identical membership.

As shown in Exhibit 11.1, the PCH hierarchy now looks like this:

- The PCH board of directors sits at the top.

- Below it is the patient care and quality enhancement committee, one of several board-level governance leadership opportunities for physicians.
- The QEC (see "The Quality Executive Committee"), one of the newly formed entities, sits parallel to the existing medical executive committee. The two committees work together, and both report directly to the patient care and quality enhancement committee.
- The other two newly formed committees, the patient safety committee and the clinical effectiveness committee, report directly to the QEC. They sit parallel to the existing clinical departments that report to the medical executive committee (MEC) (see "The Medical Executive Committee"), and they all work together.
- The various existing patient care committees all work together as well and report to the patient safety committee and the clinical effectiveness committee. In addition, they work with the existing clinical sections that report to the clinical departments that report to the MEC.
- Below the patient care committees and the clinical sections, which represent key areas of management-oriented physician leadership opportunities, sit the frontline multidisciplinary operations and clinical improvement teams. They represent some of the many operations-focused opportunities for physicians to exert leadership.

The Quality Executive Committee

The QEC's membership at PCH includes the CEO, the CNO, the CMO, the vice president for medical staff, the senior vice president for clinical operations, the CMIO, and the hospital's medical director for quality—all MDs—showing how many opportunities for physician leadership exist at the governance level under clinical integration. In addition, PCH's chief counsel is involved, as are its director of quality management and the head of medical staff services.

The Medical Executive Committee

The MEC's membership at PCH includes a president, vice president, and immediate past president, all of whom are physicians. Also, the chair of

(continued)

the credentials committee sits on the MEC, as well as the chairs of the department of anesthesia and critical care, the department of medicine, and the department of surgery, plus three physician members-at-large. Ex-officio members include the hospital's CMO (a physician), the CEO, the director of medical staff services, the PCH legal counsel, and the vice president for clinical operations.

Bird's-Eye View of Quality

The QEC's purpose is clearly defined in its charter: to provide organizational leadership and oversight in strategy and tactics relating to all dimensions of quality of care (as defined by the Institute of Medicine), plus appropriate balancing of risks and benefits when sharing quality and other data with internal and external individuals and groups.

The QEC's responsibilities are similarly spelled out in its charter. Quality-related responsibilities include the following:

- Prioritizing and monitoring implementation of the enterprise quality plan
- Overseeing the patient safety committee and the clinical effectiveness committee
- Overseeing quality initiatives
- Overseeing charter service excellence and other quality- and safety-related improvement measures
- Reviewing the hospital's quality metrics
- Holding appropriate leadership and committees accountable for performance and improvement
- Recommending allocation of funds as needed
- Communicating and interacting with the MEC around issues of quality (Exhibit 11.2). PCH has determined that communication with the MEC is an especially important channel, so the QEC is specifically charged with maintaining open and consistent channels.

The QEC is also responsible for transparency. Those duties include the following:

- Reviewing and approving policies and procedures regarding public disclosure of quality metrics and indicators, errors, and "never" events

Exhibit 11.2: Quality Issues Addressed by the MEC

Acquisition of an EKG system

Medical staff appointees to the patient safety committee and the clinical effectiveness committee

Medical staff bylaws

The medicine committee

Informed consent policies

Criteria for medical acupuncture

Nurse practitioner certification

New policies for allied health professionals regarding responsibilities of sponsoring and supervising physicians

Operations of the anesthesia and critical care services department

Dentistry criteria and delineation of privileges

Oral and maxillofacial surgery criteria and delineation of privileges

Job descriptions for nuclear medicine technologists

Family medicine criteria and delineation of privileges

Pediatric general surgery criteria and delineation of privileges

Transplant surgery criteria and delineation of privileges

Ob/gyn criteria and delineation of privileges

Update reports from the CMO

- ◆ Reviewing and approving data to be displayed internally on intranets, and publicly on the Internet
- ◆ Reviewing and recommending participation in new associations and relationships that include disclosing errors and "never" events
- ◆ Reviewing publicly reported quality information
- ◆ Undertaking new transparency initiatives as appropriate

Physician to Physician

Quality is an area where almost any physician loves to get involved. Use this motivation to give physicians a chance to try out leadership activity.
—*Jacque Sokolov, MD*

Exhibit 11.3: Committees Reporting to the Patient Safety Committee

Infection prevention and control

Transfusion

Pharmacy and therapeutics

Medication safety

QUALITY FROM THE PATIENTS' PERSPECTIVE

The patient safety committee, which reports to the quality executive committee, also holds promise for physician leadership opportunities. Its membership includes the quality management director, the medical staff vice president, the CNO, and a medical staff appointee. The committee also includes representatives from respiratory therapy, medical and surgical nursing, the laboratory, risk management, the pharmacy, facilities, and information technology.

The committee's functions, detailed in its charter, include the following:

- Responsibility for achieving elements of the enterprise quality plan
- Fostering a culture that is committed to improving patient safety
- Identifying, assessing, and recommending safety improvement initiatives, including process improvement and education
- Monitoring, measuring, and evaluating the process of institutional indicators, performance improvement teams, department monitors, and national guidelines
- Maintaining compliance with regulatory agencies
- Referring issues to other hospital and medical staff committees as needed (Exhibit 11.3)

The patient safety committee is a multidisciplinary group designed to help ensure that patient safety and service quality improvement initiatives are met. To accomplish those goals, it will further define and develop quality measurements. The patient safety committee will also focus on providing education on and promoting awareness of patient safety and quality issues and best practices. The committee will fulfill its duties by tracking strategic plans, analyzing events, providing more objective ways of tracking issues, corresponding on an ongoing basis with appropriate executives, and ensuring a culture of safety.

One goal of the patient safety committee is having facilities available that provide accurate, fact-based data. The committee has determined that relying on people's opinions to conclude observance reports is the equivalent of a "witch hunt" and that using a fact-based tracking system is more effective and efficient.

EFFECTIVENESS AS PART OF THE VALUE EQUATION

The clinical effectiveness committee (see "The Clinical Effectiveness Committee"), which also reports to the QEC, carries its own opportunities for physician leadership. Its membership includes the hospital's medical director of quality and a cochair appointed by the MEC; the hospital's CMO and CMIO; and the chairs of the departments of medicine, anesthesia and critical care, and surgery. The committee also includes a medical education representative, appointed by the hospital's graduate medical education director; the pharmacy director; the respiratory therapy director; and a nursing representative.

The committee's purpose, according to its charter, is to

- improve quality;
- establish clinical effectiveness processes;
- identify, analyze, and make recommendations for initiatives;
- ensure appropriate infrastructure to support improvement activities;
- oversee initiatives and committees; and
- communicate information.

The Clinical Effectiveness Committee

Operationally, the clinical effectiveness committee is responsible to the QEC and works alongside the MEC and the various medical staff departments.

Exhibit 11.4 shows the patient care committees that are responsible to the clinical effectiveness committee at PCH.

The clinical effectiveness committee's responsibilities are centered on implementing a process for how protocols are developed, but it does not develop them directly. The committee considered creating additional committees to report to it, including an inpatient care committee to represent heretofore overlooked inpatient units.

Exhibit 11.4: Committees Reporting to the Clinical Effectiveness Committee

Neonatal patient care

Emergency department

Critical care medicine

Radiology

Trauma operations

Preoperative oversight

Physician to Physician

What are good opportunities in an enterprise-level quality plan for new physician leaders, and which positions are better suited to experienced leaders?
—Jacque Sokolov, MD

CONCLUSION

A clinically integrated healthcare organization cannot function without a strong focus on quality—both at the enterprise level and at every level of governance, management, and operations. And that focus must incorporate the views of the personnel with the best handle on clinical quality: physicians.

While the authors have great respect for the entire program at PCH, they encourage readers to understand that one size does not fit all. Organizations are wise to carefully customize their approach to an enterprise quality plan.

Thoughts for Consideration

Does your organization have an enterprise-level quality plan? If not, why not?

Does your organization have a quality-focused department or committee that does not involve physicians in some way?

(continued)

Where do physicians have input at the governance level in your organization? Where are the physician touch points at the management level? At the operations level?

Are your organization's quality deliverables clearly defined?

Is responsibility for each of the deliverables assigned to a specific committee or department?

SUGGESTED READING

Galt, K. A., and K. A. Paschal. 2009. *Foundations in Patient Safety for Health Professionals.* Burlington, MA: Jones & Bartlett Publishers.

Nance, J. J. 2008. *Why Hospitals Should Fly: The Ultimate Flight Plan to Patient Safety and Quality Care.* Bozeman, MT: Second River Healthcare Press.

Pena, J. J., A. N. Haffner, B. Rosen, and D. W. Light. 1984. *Hospital Quality Assurance, Risk Management, and Program Evaluation.* New York: Aspen Publishers.

Pronovost, P., and E. Vohr. 2011. *Safe Patients, Smart Hospitals: How One Doctor's Checklist Can Help Us Change Health Care from the Inside Out.* New York: Plume Publishing.

Ransom, E. R., M. S. Joshi, D. Nash, and S. A. Ransom. 2008. *The Healthcare Quality Book: Vision, Strategy, and Tools.* Chicago: Health Administration Press.

Varkey, P. 2009. *Medical Quality Management: Theory and Practice,* 2nd ed. Burlington, MA: Jones & Bartlett Publishers.

CHAPTER 12

How to Assess and Select Physician Leaders

They just can't say, "I'm a physician; therefore I am a leader." But the fact is some physicians really believe they can.
—*Physician CEO*

For some reason, when it comes to making selection decisions when hiring physicians into leadership roles, what I do with other executive hiring does not work, and the whole process of trying to hire a physician leader just comes apart. There just doesn't seem to be any logical approach to the task.
—*Healthcare CEO*

My experience has been that the best clinicians get selected for management and leadership positions, and I really don't think that is always best for the organization.
—*Seasoned health system CEO*

Assessing and Selecting Physician Leaders

Assessment and selection of leaders can be improved through a process that injects as much objectivity as possible. Hiring physicians for administrative positions can be particularly challenging.

An effective process requires

- a thorough understanding of leadership,
- a well-thought-out model of selection to better understand the decision steps taken,

(continued)

> ◆ the use of leadership competencies to assess leadership skills,
> ◆ the use of solid, leadership-related personality principles, and
> ◆ a structured decision-making process for assessment and selection.

Although this chapter is a companion to Chapter 4 ("Identification of Physician Leaders"), that chapter focused on how to identify those physicians who had high potential to become effective leaders. This chapter addresses the process of assessing and selecting individuals for specific leadership positions. This may be a hiring decision involving the selection of an outside candidate for a full-time or part-time physician management or leadership position. Alternatively, the principles could be used when picking a physician to lead a task force, a committee, or another voluntary leadership role in the organization.

This chapter is founded on the belief that ample research exists to support more scientific ways of selecting leaders. The authors aim to provide a single chapter that serves as a usable and practical guide to selection.

It may be obvious to readers, but the selection of physician leaders is not that different from the selection of any other leaders; the suggestions presented in this chapter are equally applicable to all hiring situations.

Before continuing this chapter, readers are encouraged to reflect on the following questions:

◆ How should I assess candidates for leadership and management positions?
◆ How should I make a final hiring decision?
◆ What factors do I consider when choosing any leader for any task?

We believe that the selection "hit rate" or success outcome will be improved through having a deeper understanding of leadership, using a formalized selection model to guide the assessment process, using precise definitions of leadership competencies when assessing individuals, understanding the role of personality in leadership selection, and using a structured decision-making process when assessing and selecting leaders.

LEADERSHIP DEFINED

Although many books and articles expound on leadership, for the purposes of this chapter, *leadership* will be defined as follows:

A process that occurs when individuals, driven by their inborn traits (personality), practice certain behaviors (leadership competencies) that cause others to follow them in the pursuit of a vision and goals.

Leadership is a process—essentially a group of actions, operations, and functions—that brings about a result. The process involves an individual persuading others to move toward a certain goal. The process is also futuristic—it contemplates change that is designed to bring improvement. This ability to anticipate the future and prepare to make the changes needed to be successful is a hallmark of effective leadership. This concept is discussed in Chapter 5, which contrasts management and leadership. Recall that the practice of management deals mostly with day-to-day matters, while leadership involves transformation and focus on the future. When making a selection decision, hiring decision makers who understand leadership from this perspective will enhance their ability to compare and contrast candidates. While the practice of management and the practice of leadership will often overlap, the areas of assessment for positions that concern mostly day-to-day management are different from those for positions that are more leadership focused.

Leaders lead through a combination of the following factors.

Values and traits (inborn characteristics or tendencies) that shape an individual's thoughts and feelings and drive behavior. The final section of this chapter presents a personality theory (the Five Factor Model) and a psychological instrument (Hogan Assessments) to show some of the key personality traits of effective leaders—traits that form the basis of an individual's style or how an individual typically and naturally approaches people and situations. Heredity and early upbringing strongly influence these traits. Each of the five factors in the model is viewed on a continuum so that different people fall somewhere in between the extreme ends of each factor. These deep-seated characteristics guide leadership behavior.

Leadership competencies (behavioral practices) or skills that are used in leadership situations. Katz (1995) suggests that *skills* imply what leaders can accomplish, whereas *traits* imply who leaders are (their innate characteristics). Traits are mostly inborn, but skills can be learned.

Situations (contingencies) that require the behavior of leaders to match the events and the types of followers that exist. Usually called contingency leadership, this skill describes how effective leaders use different competencies in different situations. For example, an organization in a financial turnaround requires a leader with different competencies than does an organization experiencing significant growth. A chief medical officer accustomed to a fully employed physician group in a formal setting will likely have to modify his approach in a more laid-back setting with all independent physician practitioners. Goleman (2000) writes that the leaders with the best results do not rely on only one leadership style; they use multiple styles and approaches—sometimes several in a given week, seamlessly and in different measure. In addition, they are able to "switch between styles seamlessly and can also use a combination of styles depending on the business situation."

SELECTION MODEL

Logically speaking, a grounded understanding of the principles of selection leads to better hiring decisions. Exhibit 12.1 provides a useful model of the key factors that drive selection decisions. When reviewing the model, readers should ask the following questions:

- What is the mental progression that ultimately results in a hiring choice—precisely how do I make selection decisions?
- What factors drive these all-important decisions, and how do they fit into the process?

Nine key factors drive hiring decisions. These factors represent the judgments, thoughts, and feelings—some objective and some subjective—that go through

Exhibit 12.1: Selection Assessment Model

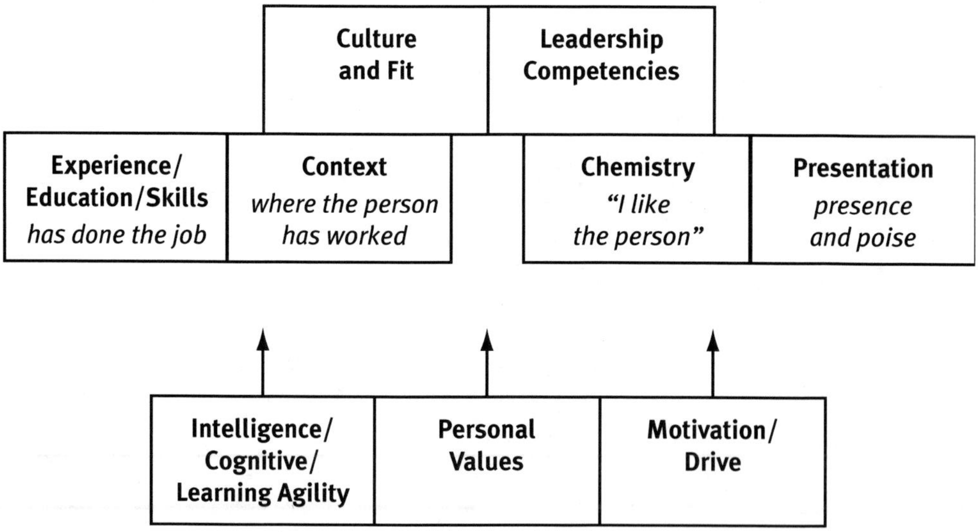

	Culture and Fit	Leadership Competencies	
Experience/ Education/Skills *has done the job*	**Context** *where the person has worked*	**Chemistry** *"I like the person"*	**Presentation** *presence and poise*

Intelligence/ Cognitive/ Learning Agility	**Personal Values**	**Motivation/ Drive**

the hiring manager's mind when making the decision to hire a candidate. When reviewing these factors, consider the significant amount of subjectivity and risk of bias involved in their evaluation.

1. **Intelligence or cognitive ability.** Intelligence and cognitive ability, whether measured or assumed, play a role in selection. Hiring decision makers make assumptions about the intelligence levels of candidates, often making comments such as "She is pretty smart" or "He is a quick learner."

2. **Personal values.** Values are those primary, deep-seated beliefs and principles that individuals consider meaningful and desirable. Individuals' values are often well developed by the time they reach their early 20s and guide their behaviors and actions.

   Values are difficult to assess and cannot be easily measured. Yet those who make hiring decisions often form strong opinions of the values of their candidates with comments such as "He is a good fit with our mission" or "Her values just fit well with us."

3. **Motivation or drive.** Motivation guides and controls behavior. In a hiring setting, it usually refers to the degree of enthusiasm, passion, or drive to perform the function of the job ("She has that 'fire in the belly' that will make her a great hire" or "He is driven to excel and achieve").

These first three factors form a person's foundation. These factors are typically innate and do not change much after age 20. They are also difficult to measure and rarely get deliberate consideration in a hiring situation. Yet taking them into account in the assessment process is important.

4. **Experience, education, and skills.** These factors are combined because typically in leadership positions, education is not considered in as much depth as experience is (e.g., a person may have a master's degree, but several years may have passed since she earned the degree or she may lack specific leadership experience). The candidate's experience is therefore weighed more heavily—especially if the candidate is already performing the job duties—and can become one of the most important factors in the hiring decision.

   Ultimately, the hiring authority concludes, "I really like what this person has done and I believe that means she can do the same for us." The authors call this the "accomplishment screen."

5. **Context.** Significant consideration is also given to where candidates have done their work—the type of organization (for-profit versus not-for-profit or academic versus community), the culture (formal versus informal or collaborative versus top-down), or the competitiveness of the market may be evaluated.

    The hiring authority may think, "I really like where this person has worked—their situation is similar to ours" or "I like the team with whom this person has worked" or "She has worked for ABC Organization, truly one of the best organizations in our industry."

6. **Chemistry.** This factor often takes the center stage in hiring decisions (see "The Role of Chemistry in Selection"), especially after meeting the candidates in person. Often this happens because the person comes from a similar background as the hiring manager (or went to the same graduate school, likes the same things, or has the same hobbies). This effect is often described as the "halo" or "similar-to-me" effect.

    Hiring authorities may conclude, "I really like her" or "I could get along quite well with this person."

7. **Presentation.** Similar to chemistry, this factor is often called *charisma* and may include a great sense of humor, positive body language, strong listening skills, a display of empathy, or good communication and interpersonal skills in general. One of the most powerful charisma factors is the ability to connect with others by getting them to identify with you. Although connectedness can be a good criterion in hiring, readers are cautioned to avoid letting this become the major factor influencing the hiring decision.

    Hiring authorities may note, "He has great presentation and speaking skills" or "She just looks like a leader" or "She has a poise about her that just shouts 'executive.'" One CEO follows this rule in hiring: "I always give them the 'restaurant test' (taking a candidate to a meal to see if he gets too relaxed) to see how they perform in that setting." (The validity of this test may be up for serious challenge.)

8. **Culture and fit.** This important factor is often overlooked because quantifying it is not easy or because most leaders are not totally forthright about descriptions of their own culture (e.g., they may describe it as collaborative when it is really more autocratic).

    Sample comments from those who make hiring decisions would be "I think she would be a great fit in our organization" or "He has the set of values that goes well in our organization."

    Note the obvious similarity of culture with the second factor, values. Values are *personal* while culture is *organizational.* But the two overlap in that individuals ideally must match their personal values with an organizational culture that embraces those values.

9. **Leadership competencies.** This factor is one of the most important and yet is shortchanged in most organizations.

   Interestingly, few hiring authorities comment specifically on leadership competencies unless their organization uses some type of formalized competency assessment tool. The descriptions rarely provide any more detail than "She is a good leader."

The Role of Chemistry in Selection

"Gut feel is used far too much in hiring decisions."

"We picked the person we all liked the best, and that was a big mistake."

"I never really thought about selection methodically until I hired some mistakes because I let chemistry drive the decision."

Chemistry and Presentation in the Hiring Process

The sad reality is that in typical hiring scenarios, factors 6 (chemistry) and 7 (presentation) take on far greater importance and weight than they should. Conversely, factors 8 (culture and fit) and 9 (leadership competencies) do not receive enough attention and focus. Despite being important and worthy of consideration, chemistry and presentation often drive the hiring decision to the exclusion of the other factors.

Readers will probably recognize this as the "halo effect," the phenomenon that occurs when an interviewer makes a generalized assumption about a candidate on the basis of chemistry and presentation—such as likability, physical looks, congeniality, dress, or deportment. Put simply, first impressions often spill over and compromise judgments about other factors.

Although chemistry and presentation do have some value, to minimize the negative impact of the halo effect, leaders should

- be aware of the power of chemistry and presentations in making judgments,
- use structured questions that are based on all of the factors in the job specification,

- use behavioral questions that require discussion of specific past job performance,
- use leadership competencies to assess candidates,
- prepare in advance for the interview, and
- involve multiple interviewers and follow-up interviews.

LEADERSHIP COMPETENCIES IN SELECTION

The 16 critical competencies (see Exhibit 12.2) set truly exceptional leaders apart from all others (Dye and Garman 2006). Whether a hiring authority uses this competency model or another one, the use of one unquestionably enhances and expands the validity and efficacy of assessing leadership in hiring.

Ranking leadership competencies relative to the leadership role in question is useful when using a competency model in selection assessment. Consider how the ranking of competencies using the Dye and Garman (2006) model might differ with regard to the following disparate vice president of medical affairs (VPMA) positions.

Position One: Medium-sized hospital in a noncompetitive market; mostly independent medical staff still organized in a fairly traditional manner. The VPMA serves mostly as a liaison with the medical staff (essentially a go-between) and manages the medical staff office functions of credentialing and medical staff affairs.

The leadership competencies that would likely have a heavier emphasis in this position would be *listening like you mean it*, *earning loyalty and trust*, and *building consensus*. While certainly all of the competencies would likely be desired, *being visionary*, *communicating vision*, or *driving results* would not likely rank as high for this type of VPMA position.

Position Two: Healthcare system composed of six hospitals in two highly competitive markets, several hundred employed physicians, and immediate plans for significant clinical integration. The leadership competencies that would have a heavier emphasis in this position would be opposite of those in position one. The higher-ranked skills would likely include *being visionary*, *communicating vision*, *cultivating adaptability*, and *building consensus*.

Position Three: Small rural hospital, the only acute care facility in a 50-mile radius; all medical staff members are employed and most are under the age of 45. The VPMA for this organization would likely need a stronger emphasis on the following leadership competencies: *listening like you mean it*, *giving feedback*, *mentoring others*, *developing teams*, *energizing staff*, *generating informal power*, *building consensus*, and *making decisions effectively*.

Exhibit 12.2: The 16 Exceptional Leadership Competencies Defined

Living by Personal Conviction

You know and are in touch with your values and beliefs, are not afraid to take a lonely or unpopular stance if necessary, are comfortable in tough situations, can be relied on in tense circumstances, are clear about where you stand, and will face difficult challenges with poise and self-assurance.

Possessing Emotional Intelligence

You recognize personal strengths and weaknesses; see the links between feelings and behaviors; manage impulsive feelings and distressing emotions; are attentive to emotional cues; show sensitivity and respect for others; challenge bias and intolerance; collaborate and share; are an open communicator; and can handle conflict, difficult people, and tense situations effectively. Emotional intelligence may often be labeled EQ, or emotional intelligence quotient.

Being Visionary

You see the future clearly, anticipate large-scale and local changes that will affect the organization and its environment, are able to project the organization into the future and envision multiple potential scenarios/outcomes, have a broad way of looking at trends, and are able to design competitive strategies and plans based on future possibilities.

Communicating Vision

You distill complex strategies into a compelling call to march, inspire and help others see a core reason for the organization to make change, talk beyond the day-to-day tactical matters that face the organization, show confidence and optimism about the future state of the organization, and engage others to join in.

Earning Loyalty and Trust

You are a direct and truthful person; are willing to admit mistakes, are sincerely interested in the concerns and dreams of others, show empathy and a generally helpful orientation toward others, follow promises with actions, maintain confidences and disclose information ethically and appropriately, and conduct work in open, transparent ways.

Listening Like You Mean It

You maintain a calm, easy-to-approach demeanor; are patient, open minded, and willing to hear people out; understand others and pick up the meaning of their messages; are warm, gracious, and inviting; build strong rapport; see through the words that others express to the real meaning (i.e., cut to the heart of the issue); and maintain formal and informal channels of communication.

(continued)

Giving Feedback

You set clear expectations, bring important issues to the table in a way that helps others hear them, show an openness to facing difficult topics and sources of conflict, deal with problems and difficult people directly and frankly, provide timely criticism when needed, and provide feedback that is clear and unambiguous.

Mentoring Others

You invest the time to understand the career aspirations of your direct reports, work with direct reports to create engaging mentoring plans, support staff in developing their skills, support career development in a nonpossessive way (will support staff moving up and out as necessary for their advancement), find stretch assignments and other delegation opportunities that support skill development, and model professional development by advancing your own skills.

Developing Teams

You select executives who will be strong team players, actively support the concept of teaming, develop open discourse and encourage healthy debate on important issues, create compelling reasons and incentives for team members to work together, effectively set limits on the political activity that takes place outside the team framework, celebrate successes together as a unit, and commiserate as a group over disappointments.

Energizing Staff

You set a personal example of good work ethic and motivation; talk and act enthusiastically and optimistically about the future; enjoy rising to new challenges; take on your work with energy, passion, and drive to finish successfully; help others recognize the importance of their work; are enjoyable to work for; and have a goal-oriented, ambitious, and determined working style.

Generating Informal Power

You understand the roles of power and influence in organizations; develop compelling arguments or points of view based on knowledge of others' priorities; develop and sustain useful networks up, down, and sideways in the organization; develop a reputation as a go-to person; and effectively affect the thoughts and opinions of others, both directly and indirectly, through others.

Building Consensus

You frame issues in ways that facilitate clarity from multiple perspectives, keep issues separated from personalities, skillfully use group decision techniques, ensure that quieter group members are drawn into discussions, find shared values and common adversaries, and facilitate discussions rather than guide them.

(continued)

Exhibit 12.2: The 16 Exceptional Leadership Competencies Defined (continued)

Making Decisions Effectively

You make decisions based on an optimal mix of ethics, values, goals, facts, alternatives, and judgments; use decision tools effectively and at appropriate times; and show a good sense of timing related to decision making.

Driving Results

You mobilize people toward greater commitment to a vision, challenge people to set higher standards and goals, keep people focused on achieving goals, give direct and complete feedback that keeps teams and individuals on track, quickly take corrective action as necessary to keep everyone moving forward, show a bias toward action, and proactively work through performance barriers.

Stimulating Creativity

You see broadly outside of the typical, are constantly open to new ideas, are effective with creativity group processes (e.g., brainstorming, scenario building), see future trends and craft responses to them, are knowledgeable in business and societal trends, are aware of how strategies play out in the field, are well read, and make connections between industries and unrelated trends.

Cultivating Adaptability

You quickly see the essence of issues and problems, effectively bring clarity to situations of ambiguity, approach work using a variety of leadership styles and techniques, track changing priorities and readily interpret their implications, balance consistency of focus against the ability to adjust course as needed, balance multiple tasks and priorities such that each gets appropriate attention, and work effectively with a broad range of people.

SOURCE: Adapted from Dye and Garman (2006).

Position Four. Successful health system that has had no turnover in its senior levels of leadership for many years, but has never had a physician in the senior ranks. The VPMA is a newly created position, and there is no consensus about the role of the job. The successful VPMA candidates for this organization would likely need a stronger emphasis on the following leadership competencies: *being visionary, communicating vision, earning loyalty and trust, mentoring others,* and *stimulating creativity.*

To make the assessment analysis more in-depth, take into account what shifts might occur with the organization over the next few years (e.g., a significant movement toward employed physicians or the full development of a clinical integration organization) to determine how adding new talent or behavior (through added leadership competencies) might shore up current deficiencies in the executive team and to try to screen out what has not worked, such as with a prior VPMA. Also, engaging in this type of analysis helps the hiring authority keep an eye on unintended side effects of asking for new capabilities (because when we ask for more strength in driving results we may also get overconfidence, unnecessary risk-taking, and arrogance). Factoring in existing team personalities and capabilities when weighting competency needs is also important. Obviously, this exercise can be taken so far that the entire process becomes cumbersome and unmanageable. But careful reflection and some form of ranking will be helpful in the final assessment of candidates.

Finally, the screening and interview process mandates that the required leadership competencies be well defined and that an assessment of each candidate's skills in those competencies be performed. These steps can be achieved through interviews, references, assessments, simulations, or a combination of all.

A note is in order regarding two of the leadership competencies in Exhibit 12.2: *living by personal conviction* and *possessing emotional intelligence*. Simply stated, these competencies are critical for *all* leaders; they always carry a high ranking. Leaders with personal conviction will be consistent in their behavior, unwavering in their drive to improve performance, and focused in their efforts. Employees are comfortable knowing their leaders will be consistent. Leaders also must have an excellent sense of who they are and how they are perceived by others. Those who are emotionally intelligent will have a keen ability to control their emotions and be socially mature. Deficiencies in these competencies also frequently cause derailment in leaders, a problem that will be discussed in detail in Chapter 15.

USING PERSONALITY IN SELECTION: THE FIVE FACTOR MODEL

Many volumes have been written about personality, and covering personality theories is beyond the scope of this book. However, one theory does prove useful in selection. The Five Factor Model suggests that five major dimensions compose personality and form the core of people in their social interactions with others.

Openness. Openness refers to how receptive a person is to different thoughts and experiences. People who have a high degree of openness are interested in learning new things; like to know how things work; have natural curiosity; and are insightful, sophisticated, and thoughtful. They are not restricted by boundaries and are strong problem solvers. They also embrace diversity, which is becoming increasingly important to today's leader.

Conscientiousness. Conscientiousness refers to a person's degree of motivation and perseverance. People who score high in this factor tend to be self-disciplined, responsible, and well organized. They face adversity well and are dependable and thorough.

Extraversion. Extraversion indicates how sociable and outgoing a person is. Persons who score high in this factor like to interact with others, are talkative and demonstrative, and reach out to others. They get along well in teams and are expressive.

Agreeableness. This factor refers to how caring for others a person is and is indicative of the degree of sensitivity shown to others. Those high in this area are cooperative and collaborative, work well with teams, and are optimistic and good-natured.

Neuroticism. Neuroticism relates to how a person reacts to pressure or difficulty. A highly neurotic person will frequently be nervous and uncertain, especially in unfamiliar situations. Those with low neurotic tendencies are calm under pressure, confident, and provide a stable presence for those around.

The Five Factors—easily remembered with the acronym OCEAN—can guide the selection of highly effective leaders in the following ways:

- **High on openness.** They come up with new and unique ideas, are adept at connecting the dots and seeing connections between events, and anticipate future trends accurately.
- **High on conscientiousness.** They approach life with a plan, present structure and reason in their work, and enjoy improving organizational performance.
- **High on extraversion.** They exhibit high energy and are comfortable being around people (even if they might have an inner feeling of introversion). They seek to be in charge and are comfortable taking unpopular stands if necessary. Others look to them for direction in a crisis.
- **High on agreeableness.** They get along with others, and they cooperate and collaborate. They see the positive in others and are not skeptical or aloof.
- **Low on neuroticism.** They are not typically tense, irritable, or moody and serve as positive and optimistic role models.

Where candidates fall on these scales can be determined through a combination of carefully crafted interviews, targeted reference discussions with former colleagues, and validated assessment tools such as the Hogan Personality Inventory. When assessing leaders, consider using the Five Factor Model as a guide but not a completely definitive indicator. The model should shape analysis as candidates are reviewed and considered, but the theory is not invincible. For example, many people who are naturally introverted are able to behaviorally exhibit strong extraverted skills that allow them to function as effective leaders.

Physician to Physician

A well-thought-out screening and selection process may be your best defense against physicians who want to armchair quarterback your selection of physician leaders.
—Jacque Sokolov, MD

USING A STRUCTURED DECISION-MAKING PROCESS

Once the recruiting process nears the end, typically two final candidates stand in the wings awaiting a decision. Often there is no clear-cut choice. To best reach the decision, hiring managers should consider the following:

1. Be certain that the process has been followed. Ensure that no part of it is given short shrift.
2. Guard against allowing chemistry and presentation to weigh too heavily.
3. Review the specific requirements set forth at the beginning of the recruitment process.
4. Review the factors in the selection model. Consider developing a scorecard (sample provided in Appendix D) to rate the two finalists.
5. Be certain the selection success factors have been covered (through behavior-based interviews, references, work samples, assessments, simulations, and input from others).

POSITION ANALYSIS

In-depth planning and analysis of the position, its role, and the required qualifications must be done before any candidate is ever interviewed. A position analysis entails breaking down a job into its component activities: its objectives and how those objectives are translated into practice, the various interrelationships within the job, the type of culture in which the job will be done, the processes involved in doing the job effectively, and the requirements needed to do the job.

The ideal selection process is circular. When the interviews are completed, the person making the final hiring decision should go back to the position analysis done at the beginning of the recruitment. The following considerations play a role in shaping the final assessment:

- What is the ultimate purpose of the position?
- What specific objectives do you want the person to accomplish?
- What activities will lead to accomplishing those objectives?

The final assessment requires that these questions be woven into the assessment of potential leaders.

CONCLUSION

Perhaps the most important and riskiest decision any leader makes is in hiring. A mistake can be disastrous and will certainly be expensive. While this determination will always carry some measure of subjectivity, the odds can be improved with a more methodical approach, the use of a well-developed assessment and selection process, and a commitment to using the tools available to help make the final evaluation.

Thoughts for Consideration

How objective are your selection processes?

Does your organization have a validated leadership competency model? If so, is it used in assessment and selection processes?

To what extent is there a methodical approach to the assessment of leaders?

SUGGESTED READING

Dye, C. F. 2002. *Winning the Talent War: Ensuring Effective Leadership in Healthcare.* Chicago: Health Administration Press.

Dye, C. F., and A. N. Garman. 2006. *Exceptional Leadership: 16 Critical Competencies for Healthcare Executives.* Chicago: Health Administration Press.

Hogan, R., and J. Hogan. 2001. "Assessing Leadership: A View from the Dark Side." *International Journal of Selection and Assessment* 9 (1–2): 40–51.

Hogan, R., and R. B. Kaiser. 2005. "What We Know About Leadership." *Review of General Psychology* 9 (2): 169–80.

Judge, T. A., D. Heller, and M. K. Mount. 2002. "Five-Factor Model of Personality and Job Satisfaction: A Meta-Analysis." *Journal of Applied Psychology* 87 (3): 530–41.

Page, L. 2010. "10 Tips to Creating a Physician-Led Integrated Care System with Advocate Health's Mark Shields." *Becker's Hospital Review.* Published September 14. www.beckershospitalreview.com/hospital-physician-relationships/10-tips-to-creating-a-physician-led-integrated-care-system-with-advocate-healths-mark-shields.html.

Srivastava, S. 2010. "Measuring the Big Five Personality Factors." Accessed February 7. www.uoregon.edu/~sanjay/bigfive.html.

READINGS ON MANAGERIAL DERAILMENT

Denton, J. M., and J. B. Van Lill. 2006. "Managerial Derailment." *XIMB Journal of Management.* Accessed October 3, 2012. www.ximb.ac.in/ximb_journal/Publications/Article-14-15.pdf.

Hogan, J., R. Hogan, and R. B. Kaiser. 2011. "Management Derailment." In *American Psychological Association Handbook of Industrial and Organizational Psychology.* Washington, DC: American Psychological Association.

Lombardo, M. M., and R. W. Eichinger. 1995. *Preventing Derailment: What to Do Before It's Too Late.* Greensboro, NC: Center for Creative Learning.

McCartney, W. W., and C. R. Campbell. 2006. "Leadership, Management, and Derailment: A Model of Individual Success and Failure." *Leadership & Organization Development Journal* 27 (3): 190–202.

CHAPTER 13

Education of Physician Leaders

Dr. Larry Smith: I have been an officer in the state medical society, have worked my way up through the elected medical staff positions in my hospital, and just completed my MBA. I am thoroughly prepared for a full-time administrative position. (*Comment: This is likely not the case. The experience and the degree may or may not be adequate to prepare for a full-time role.*)

Dr. Marjorie Redham: I learned leadership from our cardiac nursing manager. She is an excellent communicator, she manages her budget effectively, and her staff are all very loyal to her. (*Comment: With all due respect to the nursing manager, much of what was observed relates mostly to day-to-day management and may not be relevant for a broader, more strategic physician leadership job.*)

Dr. Elizabeth Williams: It really was not until my CEO asked me to chair the quality committee eight years ago that I realized what leadership was all about. (*Comment: It should be obvious that chairing a committee alone does not fully prepare one for a leadership role.*)

Dr. James Brown: Our Physician Leadership Academy prepares our docs to assume all types of leadership positions in our system. (*Comment: Attendance at courses without the requisite experiences does not fully prepare one for these roles.*)

Dr. Mary Bruce: We brought our local university's MBA faculty on-site, and our physicians are getting their MBAs from the school. It has been a simple arrangement. (*Comment: While it is laudable to do this, MBA faculty may not have the necessary content knowledge to help healthcare leaders. Moreover, gaining an MBA alone does not make one a leader.*)

> **Physician Leadership Development Program**
>
> Highly effective organizations understand the mechanics as well as the complexity of physician leadership development programs. Their programs are formalized, sufficiently funded, and carefully planned. Most important, they are multifaceted: They include various types of educational opportunities, including classroom didactics, experiential exercises, group and individual projects, mentoring, and self-study. Finally, strong physician leadership development programs recognize the contemporary concept of leadership development—essentially, that most leadership development occurs through the practice of leadership rather than through just coursework.

The opening quotes show how rudimentary many physician leadership development programs are. But if done correctly, programs may have great complexity to them. Leadership development means far more than simply taking leadership classes. This chapter explains how to set up the educational portion of a physician leadership development program.

An effective educational program should use a well-developed and validated leadership competency model to guide the content of the curriculum. This model provides a foundation on which the program can be built. Using these competencies, a successful program should identify the skills needed within physician leadership ranks and conduct ongoing assessments of existing gaps. The best programs use this information to develop customized curriculum, experiential activities, and involvement opportunities to close those gaps.

Effective programs recognize the special nature of physicians, their typical traits, and how they traditionally learn. They provide multitrack programming and have a variety of content modules for physicians to attend. Self-study programs may be offered as well as external programming, as long as all material is coordinated and linked to an overall program and objectives.

Questions to consider include the following:

- What should physicians learn in order to move into leadership positions?
- What curriculum should be created for a physician leadership development program?
- If there is a difference between management and leadership, what are the differences in educational content for courses in these topics? And what specific topics should these courses cover?
- What is the value of master's degree programs, such as in business administration or health administration, and how do they prepare a physician for management and leadership positions?

- What are the pros and cons of using outside sources for educational programming?
- In what type of educational environment do physicians best learn?
- What does contemporary leadership development theory suggest about the best ways to learn leadership?
- How much should be budgeted for physician leadership development?

PLAN FIRST

Far too many organizations wanting to develop physician leadership programs move ahead without giving adequate thought and planning to the needs and complexities involved. Some organizations put together a few courses and call it an "academy." Others send their physicians off to American College of Physician Executives (ACPE) or American College of Healthcare Executives (ACHE) programs without thinking about how these courses integrate into their needs. Other organizations offer to pay for master's degrees for some of their physicians, while others engage outside consulting companies to come on-site to present their programs.

While a written plan is a necessity to better manage and coordinate the program, the planning process itself can serve many benefits. Having a group of physicians involved in the planning and development of the leadership program can create great buy-in from the start and allow those individuals to serve as champions of the program. The planning discussions will allow the program to be better tied to both organizational and physician leadership needs. Discussions around leadership education will also provide great benefits of higher engagement and better program outcomes. One CEO who uses a physician leadership education steering council also finds that the sidebar discussions that take place around the meetings serve to keep him informed on many of the hot-button issues in his physician groups. Using a physician leadership advisory board to help guide the development of the program is not unusual.

We caution against having a single person (such as the vice president of medical affairs or director of medical education) develop the plan alone. Involving various physicians in the planning lets them learn more about leadership concepts as they discuss educational programming. The planning process also provides additional opportunities to discern the differences between management and leadership (as discussed in Chapter 5). The discussion process around plan development also gives all participants the chance to fully explore the many ways leaders are educated. Involving several nonphysician leaders (ideally those with expertise in adult and contemporary leadership education) in the planning process is wise. Ideally, development of the plan should follow a typical strategic planning process and provide for consensual development of goals and objectives. Consider the guide in Exhibit 13.1.

TRANSITION OPPORTUNITIES

One of the most important considerations in a physician leadership development program is the transition from clinical care to administrative roles. This process is further complicated by the fact that many physicians will remain active clinically, even if on a part-time basis. "Special Considerations for the Transition from Clinical to Administrative Duties" provides some of the key questions and factors to be considered in the planning process.

Special Considerations for the Transition from Clinical to Administrative Duties

- Is the physician running away from the burdens (e.g., insurance, declining income, night call) of clinical practice? If so, how does this factor into the motivation to learn leadership and management?
- If the motivation to move into an administrative position is to "change the world," how can this lofty goal be tempered?
- Does the educational program deal with the culture shock that comes with a departure from clinical practice?
- Should most clinicians be encouraged to "wean off" clinical care rather than make a sudden shift?
- How can the educational program offerings help physicians deal with the emotional aspects of moving into administration?

TRAINING AND EDUCATION CONTENT SUGGESTIONS

The brief overview in Exhibit 13.2 suggests some content areas that would be covered in a typical curriculum. Note the differentiation between management-oriented and leadership-oriented content. A good program will provide many choices and have a multitrack curriculum.

Exhibit 13.1: Developing a Physician Leadership Education Program

Mission and Objectives

♦ Why is the organization developing this program?
♦ Does the plan address involvement of physicians in management and leadership positions?
♦ What are the desired outcomes of a physician leadership education and involvement program?

Analysis of Current Programs

♦ What leadership education do current physicians have or need?
♦ Do we use a leadership competency model to drive our program content?
♦ What types of physician leaders currently participate (and will this change)?
  - Full-time clinician who remains full-time in clinical practice but plays some role in leadership (e.g., medical staff–elected role, part-time division chief, or medical director or physician-in-charge)
  - Full-time clinician dropping some clinical practice hours to move into an administrative role
  - Physician assuming a management role
  - Physician assuming a leadership role
  - Full-time physician executive
  - Physician leader being developed for a different role in the future

Strategy Formulation

♦ How will the plan be developed so that education can cover the various types of physician leaders?
♦ How much of the curriculum will be didactic?
♦ How much of the didactic curriculum will be taught by internal resources versus external resources?
♦ To what extent will the programming provided through organizations such as ACHE and ACPE be used?
♦ How will master's degree programs be used in the plan?
♦ Who can attend the program? (See Chapter 4 on the process for identifying physician leaders.)
♦ How will the program be evaluated?

Execution Through Clear Objectives

♦ Are most of our physician leaders in the latter stages of their careers? Do we need to get younger participants? Should a formal succession plan for physician leadership be developed?
♦ Should the principles of clinical integration be key components of the program? And if so, how sensitive will it be to introduce them?
♦ Do we need to prepare for more full-time physician leaders in the organization?

(continued)

Program, Curriculum, Budget, Procedures, Written Plan, and Follow-Up

- Who will develop the specific curriculum?
- Who will assemble the faculty? Will faculty be from inside or outside the organization or a mix?
- Does the program have an adequate budget?
- How will meaningful experiential activities be built into the program?

IMPORTANT CONSIDERATIONS

Leadership Through Experiences

One of the most overlooked aspects of development is the need for experiential exercises. Learners need to practice what they learn. Two types of experiential exercise are critical—crucible experiences and growth through experience.

Crucible experiences. Robert Thomas (2008) wrote, "Leaders learn how to lead from experience. Formal training can help, but it's no substitute for learning on, and off, the job." All classroom programs and rich didactic curricula are wasted if physicians do not have the chance to put the principles into practice. Interestingly, physicians train exactly this way—yet many organizations rely solely on classroom courses to produce physician leaders and managers.

> To leverage experiences that involve reversal, people should be comfortable with self-observation and self-regulation and be capable of coping with adversity and exercising sympathy.
> —*Robert J. Thomas (2008)*

A crucible experience is one in which an individual is tested, stretched, or challenged by something real. The experiences could take place at work or in other settings. Some leaders have honed great skills through taking on leadership roles in churches and other outside organizations. Crucible experiences can take place when leaders are put into situations they have not confronted before. Thomas (2008) suggests that there are three types of crucible experiences:

1. New territory: when someone is placed in a different role or position with different skill set demands, essentially dealing with the unknown
2. Reversal: when there has been a loss or failure
3. Suspension: a situation that requires an extensive time of reflection or deliberation

Exhibit 13.2: Introduction to Physician Leadership

Leadership Education

Leadership theory
Leadership competencies
Organizational vision
Emotional intelligence
Managing change
Creative planning techniques for corporate innovation and growth

Management Training

Budgets, financial forecasting
Planning and contingency variables
Staffing and scheduling, management controls
Decision making
Delegating
Operations management
Human resources management
Conflict resolution
Use of roles when working as a team
Communication process
Identifying one's predominant decision-making style
Recognizing commitment levels (one's own and others') to the organization's goals
Explaining how planning adds to an organization's goals
Organizational structure and organizational design options

Business Training

Healthcare 101: the healthcare delivery system and its component parts
Clinical integration models
Healthcare finance
Health law
Marketing and planning principles
Information technology

Personal Training and Education

Time management
Office management
Personal management
Balancing work and life
Managing personal health

Some physicians are motivated to move into leadership and management roles because of crucible experiences. Some have a strong motivation to fix something as the result of some obstacle, often an organizational one, while others seem to gravitate toward leadership roles because of a series of struggles that alter their career motives.

Growth through experience. Michael Lombardo and Robert Eichinger wrote about the need to allow experience to finish what nature starts. In their excellent book *The Leadership Machine* (2002), they posit that "skill development is reported as 75 percent to 90 percent learned on the job." Their research suggests that development occurs only when there is something at stake.

If you ask seasoned leaders what contributed most to their growth, many would name specific experiences. An ideal leadership development program should be a combination of coursework and experiential learning.

Physician to Physician

There are two extremes when it comes to the use of on-the-job training (OJT) for physician leaders. One involves no formal training and only OJT, and the other involves extremely structured leadership training concurrent with OJT. OJT—through apprenticeships and traditional mentoring—was predominant for developing physician leaders historically. But structured education and leadership development programs are now the norm. These do not diminish the importance of OJT, but finding a successful physician leader who has not had some type of formalized training is rare.
—Jacque Sokolov, MD

One distinctive area of experience-based learning for physicians involves working within teams. As discussed in Chapter 1, physicians by nature are independent, and much of their work is often done in a solo capacity. Working in teams frequently requires ample practice for physicians. Educational focus should be given to how teams are best formed and how they are best managed.

In developing physician leadership and management development programs, organizations must build in experiential opportunities. This can be achieved through different assignments, including leading a task force, appointment to a board committee, heading a start-up for a new program or service, or managing a turnaround.

HOW DO SMART PEOPLE LEARN?

Harvard professor Chris Argyris proposed the concept of single-loop and double-loop learning (Smith 2001). Single-loop learning is akin to a thermostat set to a specific temperature; the thermostat makes an automatic adjustment when the temperature is not at that figure. By contrast, double-loop learning would involve reflection about what the ideal temperature should be, based on different variables. In a single-loop learning situation, memorization is effective; adjustments need not be considered. By contrast, in a double-loop learning situation, recognition that there are multiple and changing variables does not allow for rote responses. As Argyris put it, this system "may then lead to an alteration in the governing variables and, thus, a shift in the way in which strategies and consequences are framed" (Smith 2001).

> Learning is a function of how people reason about their own behavior. Yet most people engage in defensive reasoning when confronted with problems. They blame others and avoid examining critically the way they have contributed to problems.
> —Chris Argyris (1991)

A final comment is warranted about the inclusion of nonphysicians in leadership development programs. Although there is merit to the belief that "We will be shaping the future healthcare system together, so we should learn and develop together," initial exposure to physician management and leadership ideally is accomplished in the safety of a physician-only audience.

Physician to Physician

Physician leaders need to learn how to collaborate with nonphysician leaders—there will always be a blend of physician and nonphysician leaders running the clinically integrated organization.
—Jacque Sokolov, MD

CONCLUSION

Developing an effective leadership and management development program for physician leaders is not easy. Significant planning and adequate resources must be provided. Doing it right costs money. Careful development of synchronized plans and curricula that include many well-established programs for hands-on experiences, exposure, and involvement will go far to ensure a strong program.

Thoughts for Consideration

Does your organization have a written plan for physician leadership development and involvement?

Do you recognize yourself in any of the comments on the first page of this chapter?

What will it take to change that attitude?

How does your organization integrate customized, internal leadership and management imperatives with the broader content structure provided by outside organizations like ACHE and ACPE?

Does your leadership development program include both didactic and experiential learning opportunities?

Do you have a formal structure for preparing physicians for the culture shock of leaving clinical practice?

SUGGESTED READING

Kaplan, A. S., E. Porter, and L. Klobnak. 2012. "Creating a Strategy-Based Physician Leadership Development Program." *The Physician Executive* 38 (1): 22–25.

Outlaw, D. 2010. "Division Chiefs: Challenges and Successes: Transitioning into Physician Leadership Roles." *Advances in Business-Related Scientific Research Journal.* www.absrc.org/ABSRJ_Outlaw.pdf.

Thomas, R. J. 2008. *Crucibles of Leadership: How to Learn from Experience to Become a Great Leader.* Boston: Harvard Business Press.

CHAPTER 14

Case Examples of Physician Leadership Development Programs

There are a lot of ways to do this. It is not just about getting a few docs to get their MBAs.

—CEO of eastern health system

Physician leadership development touches all aspects of our physician world. Everything we do with physicians has some physician leadership development aspect.

—Longtime physician executive

Until we fully realized that we needed to have all of our physicians—even those who were not in leadership positions—engaged in some manner in the direction setting of our organization, we just had passengers on our bus. When we got them engaged, the bus came alive. We have seen some great successes the past couple of years.

—Midwestern health system CEO

Physician leadership development is about so much more than just offering a collection of courses or paying for some MBAs. It involves interaction with physicians at all levels, providing information about the organization's direction and listening to those physicians' thoughts and concerns. It might include mentoring and coaching as well as taking time to encourage younger physicians who might exhibit leadership skills and interests to get more involved. It comprises physician recognition programs and developing strong two-way communications programs. Organizations can help physicians learn fundamental skills—such as making decisions, running meetings, and providing basic human resources functions—that may be useful to them in their practices. And it involves having an effective conflict-management program.

REORGANIZING THE PHYSICIAN LEADERSHIP GROUP

This chapter provides specific examples of how different organizations are approaching physician leadership and physician involvement.

CENTRAL MAINE HEALTHCARE AND THE CENTRAL MAINE MEDICAL GROUP

With thanks to Laird Covey, president, Central Maine Medical Center, and David Frum, president, Bridgton Hospital and Rumford Hospital

Central Maine Healthcare (CMHC), a leading integrated healthcare system composed of four hospitals and a large multispecialty provider group, has annual net revenues of approximately $500 million. The multispecialty practice, Central Maine Medical Group (CMMG), has approximately 375 providers in 16 communities across central, coastal, and western Maine. CMMG includes 36 medical and surgical specialties and is an employment model. Over the past few years, CMHC has focused on developing a new model for its physician leadership.

Evolution of the Need for Change

Historically, the medical staff structures in place in the four CMHC system hospitals were no different from other systems with a voluntary model of medical staff leadership. Like many organizations, though, CMHC knew this structure had problems. It perpetuated a significant disconnect in needed versus realized medical staff leadership. It also created inherently flawed dynamics regarding how important decisions were made (think of the traditional saying that a 10:1 vote in a medical staff is called a "tie").

CMHC had a long-standing commitment to the employment model, and that commitment created further disconnects with the traditional medical staff structure. As the employment model grew, the voluntary medical staff structure realized less connection and less participation within system decision making (essentially, two parallel structures existed, and neither was working optimally). In late 2012, the system intentionally began a search for a new model, given that the employment model had reached its tipping point and thus created significant need for a new medical staff leadership structure. At the time CMHC was searching for a structure, it could not find one to replicate. So, with counsel, it conceptualized its own model.

The system remained committed to the employment model and wanted to retain some level of engagement with remaining voluntary medical staff leadership. To begin, the system created a new role—medical group president—that also carried the title of medical staff president. The system retained its medical executive committee (MEC) but integrated employed and voluntary medical staff and nonvoting key members from administration, the board, and nursing. Majority membership on the MEC was composed of appointed rather than elected leaders. Then the system created divisional chief roles to whom section leaders would report. The chief role is compensated (50 percent of worked time). Four chiefs work in the largest hospital (and provide regional leadership in certain specialties), and one chief sits in each of the smaller, rural facilities (25 percent of worked time in smaller facilities).

Medical Staff Leadership Today: Lessons Learned

Living in two parallel worlds was not working for anyone. Admittedly, a commitment to this new structure may well have created greater angst in the nonemployed members of the medical staff. But no matter what belief CMHC had going into this change, it underestimated the time, training, and support resources its new medical leaders would require. While the chiefs are dedicating 25 to 50 percent of their time toward leadership, other demands compete for their attention. Yet CMHC knew that if the chiefs spent more time as leaders, the perception that these leaders were active members of the medical staff might be weakened. The investment made in this leadership structure was large. But as CMHC committed to a new model and new way to structure its medical staff, it saw the expense as a necessary investment.

The true integration of medical staff leaders, administration, and other key constituencies has driven new and improved results. CMHC feels it is still too early to do a full analysis, but the organization knows adjustments will be made and believes its new structure is taking root and working.

Considerations for the future will include compensation of section leaders, support resources for chiefs, succession planning, and training of new and future medical staff leaders. The interrelation between the medical staff and board has never been stronger. The two groups recently had their first joint quality meeting and saw high levels of engagement. While CMHC knows many peer organizations are struggling with provider disengagement, its quarterly primary and specialty care forums generate high attendance levels and active participation (and, importantly, include social time). CMHC realizes what is still to come: the challenges of evolving from four separate medical staffs to one, yet retaining local decision making.

HEARTLAND HEALTH

With thanks to Mark Laney, MD, president and CEO, Heartland Health, and Martha Davis, director, Organizational Consulting

Heartland Health is a successful integrated health delivery system that includes Heartland Regional Medical Center, Heartland Clinic, Heartland Foundation, and Community Health Improvement Solutions. Heartland Health is the leading provider in a 21-county area of northwest Missouri, northeast Kansas, and southeast Nebraska. Heartland has been recognized in many ways for its quality and service to its community, including winning the 2009 Baldrige National Quality Award.

Physician Involvement and Leadership

Heartland Health was committed to building a culture that brought the physician's voice clearly to the strategic table. In the early 2000s, Heartland built a structure conceived to bring physician leadership to the service line domain. The structure had some of the earmarks of the Mayo dyad model (see "The Dyad Model") but customized for Heartland. In 2012, a new organizational structure was formalized that included physician leadership at every level in the organization—from the C-suite through all of its entities, service lines, and units. In this structure, physicians serve in full- or part-time roles as partners to administrative leaders. This new dyad structure was established to ensure Heartland's readiness for healthcare transformation.

The Dyad Model

The dyad model is based on Dr. W. J. Mayo's precept, "The best interest of the patient is the only interest to be considered, and in order that the sick may have the benefit of advancing knowledge, union of forces is necessary . . . . It has become necessary to develop medicine as a cooperative science" (Zismer and Brueggeman 2010). The dyad model of leadership provides for a physician and a nonphysician to jointly lead and manage an area.

The Dyad Model (continued)

Physician manager/leader

Focus on:
• Clinical aspects
• Physician coaching
• Quality and patient safety

Nonphysician leader/manager

Focus on:
• Finance and budget
• Business operations
• System management

Overlapping responsibilities

• Equal in org structure
• Joint accountability
• Joint meetings
• Mutual interdependence
• Strategic partners

The model has taken several forms but typically includes the following:

• A pairing of two managers/leaders, one a physician who practices clinically some portion of time (but who has had some management and leadership education) and the other a full-time business or administrative individual
• Decisions made jointly
• Joint oversight of an integrated service line (e.g., cancer, neuro, heart services, orthopedics) or a business unit (e.g., outpatient facility, inpatient hospital, area of a hospital facility, regional primary care program, employed physician network)

The dyad model may be reflected at one or more levels of the organization; in some forms, administrative vice presidents are paired with physicians, and in others, the model is only applied at a service line or departmental level (such as the department of radiology or the lab).

Initial Work

Long recognizing the need for physician alignment, Heartland instituted a quality management board (QMB) to coalesce physicians and administrators around quality and performance improvement. In the board's early stages, some physicians attended courses offered by the Advisory Board Physician Leadership Academy, while others sought development through external conferences, such as ones offered by the American College of Physician Executives. Yet most physicians learned through their activity on the QMB.

> We use the Mayo dyad model to create what I call "healthy friction." We have to emphasize in that pairing, it's not that one physician is solely looking at things operationally, and one looking at things solely clinically. They have to work together.
> —*Bryan Mills, president and CEO, Community Health Network (Hennagir 2012)*

Heartland's second-tier leadership development effort was more robust. The original members of QMB—both administrators and physicians—were in the first cohort of the Advisory Board's local healthcare fellowship program. As more formal training was offered, this investment helped physicians think more broadly and more critically about the challenges and strategies leaders faced in achieving Heartland's vision and strategic priorities.

In 2009, the board of directors replaced the retiring CEO with a physician executive (Mark Laney, MD), which sent a new signal to the medical staff that a physician voice would be embedded into future decisions. From the beginning, the new CEO partnered closely with the chief operating officer, and a new commitment to a dyad structure was launched and modeled in a highly visible way.

Progress

Following this foundational work, the organization spent many months finalizing role descriptions and expectations, broadcast the new roles internally and externally to attract top-tier physician leader candidates, and completed a new organizational structure designating the new dyad relationships. At the same time, Heartland organized service lines around the patient continuum of care. The organization interviewed and selected physician leaders who commanded the respect of their colleagues for their clinical skills and also for their values, behaviors, and other leadership characteristics.

Going Forward

Many of the new physician leaders have already invested in leadership learning, but Heartland plans to make an additional investment in leadership development in the following ways:

- Those physician leaders who have not completed the Advisory Board fellowship credential will be enrolled as a priority in the next academy cohort offered locally.
- All new dyad leaders will be invited to the quarterly leadership development institutes and similar programs. Physician leaders may also attend any future offerings through the Advisory Board Physician Leadership Academy.
- A learning cohort for the service line and dyads will be offered.
- Heartland's curriculum will be based on its leadership competency model, illustrated in Exhibit 14.1.

PROMEDICA HEALTH SYSTEM

With thanks to Randy Oostra, president and CEO, ProMedica; Lee Hammerling, MD, president of ProMedica Physicians; and David James, MD, chief quality and integration officer

Established in 1986, ProMedica is a locally owned, nonprofit healthcare organization serving northwest Ohio and southeast Michigan. ProMedica has nearly 4 million patient visits annually and is composed of nearly 1,900 physicians, including more than 350 employed physicians and 100 extenders overseeing 310 facilities in 27 counties with 2,269 licensed inpatient beds and more than 70,000 inpatient discharges. ProMedica is one of the leading integrated healthcare organizations in the United States.

Several years ago ProMedica decided to deal with physician leadership development and involvement through more of a cafeteria-style approach. Rather than relying on a single method, the organization decided that multiple strategies and tactics would best help them. As a result, ProMedica has enrolled many of its physicians in a variety of ways and has become a model physician-centric organization. One indication of its success is that its physician engagement and satisfaction scores went up during EMR implementation.

ProMedica used the following precepts to guide its strategy.

A physician executive manager career path. Although most health systems have virtually no pipeline for physician leaders, ProMedica knows that the demand

Exhibit 14.1: Heartland Health Dyad Leadership Development

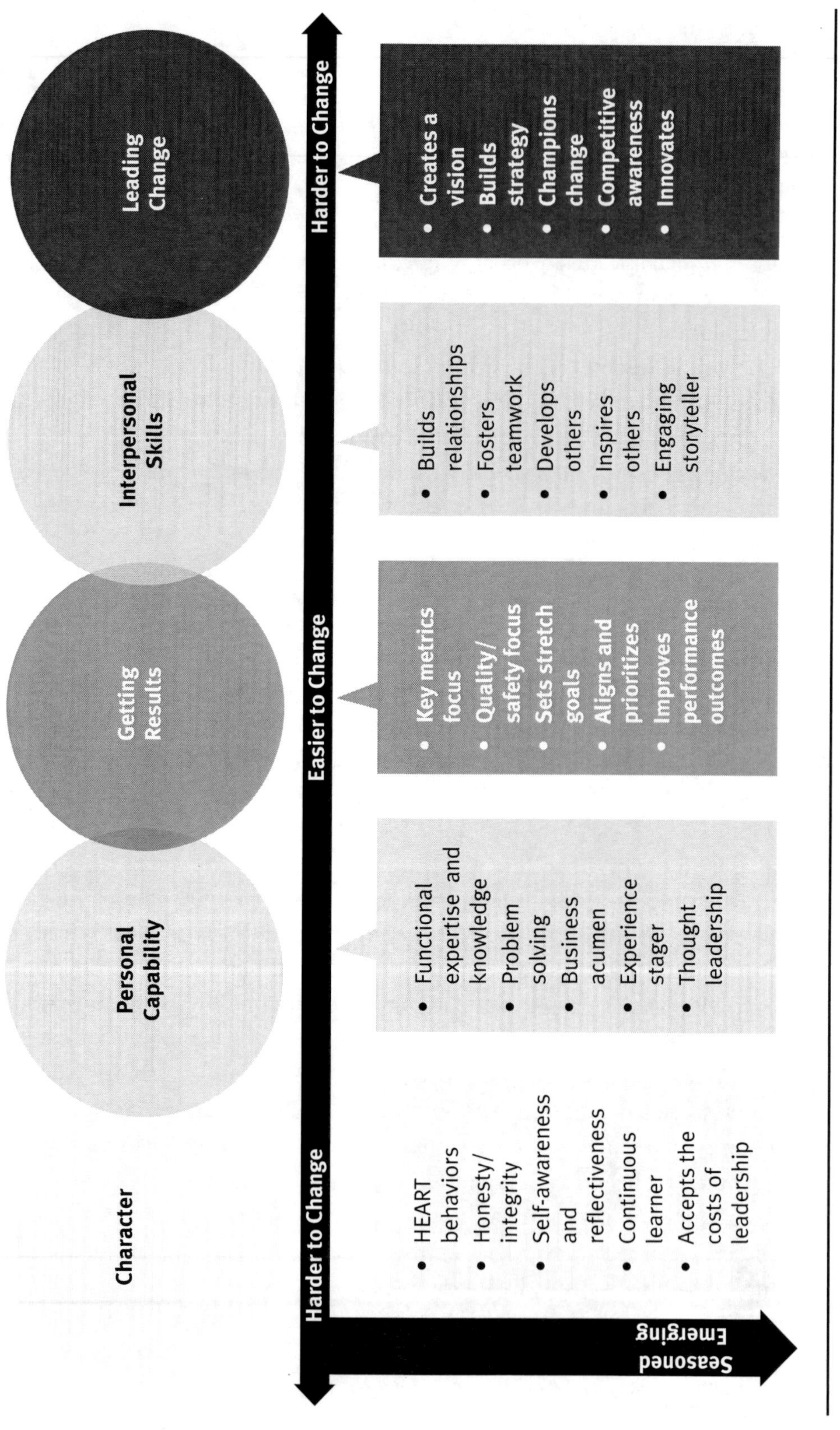

Character

- HEART behaviors
- Honesty/ integrity
- Self-awareness and reflectiveness
- Continuous learner
- Accepts the costs of leadership

Personal Capability

- Functional expertise and knowledge
- Problem solving
- Business acumen
- Experience stager
- Thought leadership

Getting Results

- Key metrics focus
- Quality/ safety focus
- Sets stretch goals
- Aligns and prioritizes
- Improves performance outcomes

Interpersonal Skills

- Builds relationships
- Fosters teamwork
- Develops others
- Inspires others
- Engaging storyteller

Leading Change

- Creates a vision
- Builds strategy
- Champions change
- Competitive awareness
- Innovates

Harder to Change — Easier to Change — Harder to Change

Seasoned / Emerging

and requirement for expert physician leader capability is and will continue to greatly outstrip supply. As the organization studied its options for sourcing, it knew it would have to hire from the outside or develop leaders from within. ProMedica concluded, as many organizations have, that the wise option was to develop from within. ProMedica saw as its emerging talent pool physicians who have been identified through multiple systematic avenues as possessing the characteristics required for various management and leadership positions within the organization. The organization determined several years ago that it needed to actively manage succession planning and cultivation through the office of organizational development.

Overlapping operational responsibilities. ProMedica adopted a dyad model of management in many areas of the organization. It based its decision on a growing paradigm in integrated delivery system models that medical and administrative operations should be equally responsible for the ultimate organizational goal of producing value for patients and payers. ProMedica ensured that the culture was one in which administrative operational responsibilities, while distinct from medical, must nevertheless be aligned with medical operations, and vice versa. Their structure was based on

1. an administrative comanager responsible for infrastructure, revenue management, expense management, capital planning, staffing, accounting reporting, feasibilities, supply chain, and support services;
2. a physician executive functioning as one side of a common coin with an administrative counterpart; and
3. a dyadic structure replicated at all levels of operational management physician group councils, medical staffs, and boards. The program is fully funded by the system, and the content is rigorous and focused.

Well-defined areas of medical operational responsibility. ProMedica determined specifically which areas should come under the direction of physician managers and leaders. It concluded the following areas required some amount of physician input and guidance into decision making:

1. Quality assurance: outcomes, evidence-based best practices, organizational transparency, and managing physician performance
2. Network integration: ensuring input from all group members, network utilization, physician relations, and outcome-driven culture
3. Managing provider productivity: contract modeling and negotiation for retention
4. Regulatory compliance: fraud and abuse, Stark, telemedicine, and e-health

5. Managing physician-driven clinical resource usage and allocation
6. Lean clinical workflow management
7. Six Sigma management of process and clinical variation among providers.

This new model of physician-driven operational management (see Exhibit 14.2) was adopted to enhance ProMedica's success and called for substantially advanced job requirements, which were served in part by the development of its Physician Executive Management Academy.

Physician Executive Management Academy. ProMedica established its Physician Executive Management Academy (PEMA) to provide a formalized education in the skills, education, and hands-on training required to develop an ongoing supply of highly capable physician managers. System leadership declared that all physician director, management, and executive positions would be operational in nature and evidence of substantive formal education in medical management would be heavily weighted, if not required, for candidates for those positions. The goal was to build a superior in-house bull pen of qualified and interested physician executives to fill the future needs for the health system.

The PEMA was set up as a formal partnership with the American College of Physician Executives (ACPE) for course content and delivery, and the faculty was to provide on-site courses four to six times per year. Course selections count toward continuing medical education and certification with ACPE; the program also provides graduate credit at the University of Toledo. In keeping with the belief that leadership is best learned through experience, the leadership group is required to work on one to two system project selections with return on investment during the program. Finally, and perhaps different from most other physician leadership development programs, the group was to include nonphysician managers and administrators to foster the operational dyad approach.

Sample content in the PEMA included the following:

◆ Governance
◆ Medical informatics
◆ Physician in management
◆ Disruptive behavior
◆ Physician–hospital relations
◆ High stakes negotiation
◆ Practice management
◆ Change leadership
◆ Healthcare finance
◆ Healthcare law

Exhibit 14.2: ProMedica Physician Executive Management Development

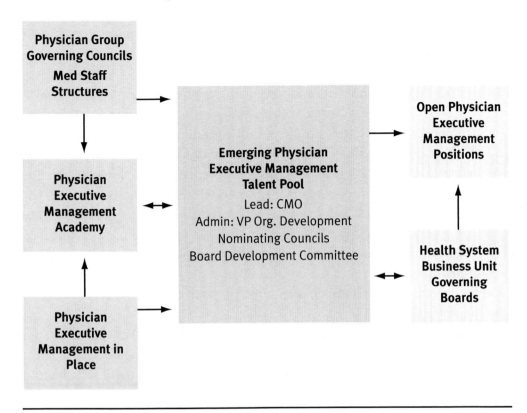

- Lean/Six Sigma
- Medical staff officer leadership

Participants in the PEMA include a defined number of physicians and nonphysician managers and executives. Each must be invited to apply, and candidates are selected on the basis of interviews, data from the emerging talent pools, and the results of the succession planning processes.

Physician leadership succession planning. ProMedica also conducted an annual review of physicians who had been involved in council governance and determined performance, development needs, and opportunities. This review formed the basis of annual succession planning, talent pool identification, and recommendations for the emerging talent pool.

Once physician leaders were moved into the succession planning program, ProMedica determined ways to integrate them with acute care executive teams in strategic and management planning; got them actively engaged with chief medical officers or vice presidents of medical affairs to shift major areas of focus to clinical operations using Lean or Six Sigma and clinical workflow management by service lines or units; aligned requirements for key medical staff positions to mirror those of physician executive requirements in the system; got system leadership to overtly reinforce that these positions and activities are developmental toward any future management activities; and perhaps most important, conducted annual performance reviews and individual succession planning with the physician leaders.

ProMedica also determined that it needed to continue to support the growth and further development of its current physician executives. It did this by taking all existing physician executive positions and "operationalizing" them around the direct management and engagement of providers and staff in quality, service, operational efficiency, network integration, medical informatics, and similar issues. The organization also developed ways for the physician executives to become actively integrated with the management of the employed physician network practices, physician governance, and medical staffs to cultivate emerging talent. Moreover, ProMedica also provided significant support for ongoing education and training in medical management areas of developmental or system need and also did annual succession and career development planning with each physician executive and his reporting structure.

A final unique way in which ProMedica enhanced physician leadership and engagement was to increase the number of physicians on all its boards and to select physicians for those boards on the basis of their areas of expertise and contribution to that board or subcommittee. Those physician members receive formal training in governance and fiduciary roles.

In addition to the above program, ProMedica has also engaged physicians as executives both in traditional management structures and comanagement arrangements. They have involved hundreds of physicians in formal strategic planning exercises and multiple informal discussions. In fact, since 2009, ProMedica leadership has held more than 19,000 meetings with groups of physicians, small and large.

ProMedica's success to date has been remarkable. It has completed its first PEMA and has several physician leaders ready to fill opportunities; plans for a second PEMA program are under way. Another positive is that the PEMA program is recognized as credit toward a master's degree at the University of Toledo, which will allow many physicians to earn their degree locally. As ProMedica's chief quality and integration officer Dr. David James stated, "The major reason we have been successful is the high level of communication that has taken place. I also think some of it is structural, in that we have committed to the development of strong physician leadership. We are poised to break out. And I would add that I have been managing the anxiety of the nonphysician executives by telling them, 'You don't have to worry—there is plenty for you to do. We need you badly.'"

MANY HOSPITALS AND HEALTH SYSTEMS

With thanks to many CEOs and other leaders

As simple as it might seem, one successful way of enhancing physician leadership is to bring physician leaders to *every* senior leadership team meeting, allowing physicians to become full-fledged members of the senior team. Organizations that have paid part-time or full-time chairs or chiefs often invite physicians to their meetings. Smaller organizations may designate certain physicians to become regular members and attendees of senior leadership meetings.

What are the keys to success using this approach? Physicians must be fully vested in the total leadership of the organization. Organizations must recognize that physicians need to be *part of the entire process*, not just asked for their opinions.

Thoughts for Consideration

Does your organization understand that practically any successful efforts made toward involving physicians, engaging them in leadership, and giving them more opportunities for leadership and management development will enhance their buy-in?

Is your organization guilty of waiting for the "perfect" educational program to get physicians more engaged?

Do your medical staff feel engaged in the development of their leadership and involvement programs?

Has your organization considered the dyad model of management/leadership?

Does your medical staff governance structure look outdated?

SUGGESTED READING

Brueggemann, J. G., and D. K. Zismer. 2008. "Physician Autonomy in Integrated Health Systems." *Group Practice Journal*, October.

Fink, J. N., and S. T. Hartzel. 2010. "From Acquisition to Integration: Transforming a Hospital into an ACO." *Healthcare Financial Management* 64 (10): 90–98.

Zismer, D. K., and P. E. Person. 2008. "The Future of Management Education and Training for Physician Leaders." *The Physician Executive* 34 (6): 44–46, 48.

Zismer, D. K., P. E. Person, and R. Aggarwal. 2009. "Finding Economic Leverage in the Fully Integrated Health System Model." *Group Practice Journal*, May.

CHAPTER 15

Avoiding Derailment

For some reason, when a physician leader fails, it seems worse than when other leaders fail.
    —Midwestern health system CEO

What got you to the dance may not get you home.
    —A seasoned hospital vice president of medical affairs

Selecting the wrong physician leader or manager can result in significant disaster. Many physician leaders are promoted from within because of their personal relationships with the physicians in the organization. They have often worked in part-time leadership roles and may have served as elected leaders of the medical staff. As such, terminating the physician leader can cause serious contention. And because of the special bond that exists among physicians, even those physician leaders who are recruited from outside the community will have special ties to each other. Moving physician leaders out of their positions is often the most difficult decision executives have to make. The authors contend that steps need to be taken to significantly reduce the chance that this might happen. Knowing more about derailment and the causes surrounding leadership hiring mistakes can head off possible danger.

As discussed in Chapter 1, physicians are among the most driven and high-achieving individuals in society. As a group, they typically are highly intelligent and do well. Physician leaders are often more sophisticated and present potentially serious problems when they have to be terminated. The quotes at the beginning of this chapter suggest that the decision to terminate a physician has far-reaching implications. Physicians are part of a guild, and when guild members are challenged, the other members close ranks around them. And typically when any executive is terminated, the reason is often shrouded in secrecy or by a confidentiality agreement. When physician leaders are terminated, this can lead to rampant speculation among the guild (medical staff). Even if the reasons for termination are nonclinical, some physicians will raise the patient care cloak and protest. As Keckley (2012a) stated, "Medicine is different than any other profession: The rigor of training, expectations of perfection, the trust conferred is perhaps unmatched by no other occupational group."

Moreover, because of the complexity of what physician leaders do, determining that a hiring mistake has been made takes much longer. The role is often poorly defined, making it tougher for a physician who is promoted into a position for which he is not well suited or fully prepared. This is not the case with other executives, whose roles are much more specifically prescribed (e.g., the number-two finance person, the assistant director of nursing, or a chief operating officer). Individuals in these other positions have had the chance to spend time in under-study positions, while the physician leaders have spent time in clinical care. Finally, physician executive salaries are often the second-highest in an organization, which can lead to expensive severance arrangements. Executives must be ever mindful of the special challenges involved in physician leader terminations.

Studying the causes of these terminations can help prevent them in the future. Clearly, some of the problems are caused by poor assessment and selection processes (covered in Chapter 12), and readers are advised to adopt the principles presented there. Some problems occur as the result of poorly defined expectations or changing job demands. Yet many are caused by the inability of physician executives to detect common derailment factors. This chapter presents a methodical review of all of these factors to help executives be diligent in their talent management.

INTRODUCTION TO MANAGERIAL DERAILMENT

The concept of managerial derailment has been discussed for almost 30 years. While many studies have focused on the issue, researchers at the Center for Creative Leadership brought the ideas front and center. The best definition may be as follows: "It's not starting well that counts, but ending well. Leadership 'derailment' occurs when a leader, who had the ability and opportunity to accomplish more, ends up fired or demoted or simply fails to succeed at the level for which he or she was called and gifted" (Webber 1998).

Some readers may quickly leap to the conclusion that this describes the "Peter Principle" made famous by the book of the same name (Peter and Hull 1969). The idea of the Peter Principle is that individuals who begin somewhat successfully in their careers eventually are promoted one level higher than their level of competence. The *Dilbert* comic and the popular television show *The Office* have reinforced that theory. However, consider the following points. The Peter Principle did not focus specifically on leadership but addressed all levels of employees in an organization. The research done to support the concept was not as robust as that which supports the study of managerial derailment. And of course, *Dilbert* and *The Office* are entertainment, not research. Finally, our discussions in this book center on multifaceted leadership issues involving physicians and the complex organizations known as hospitals.

Derailment focuses on leaders and managers who have already been effective. They have a track record of success, perhaps in another job or in their current job. But something changes, and the leader or manager begins to derail. Many physicians who have had a stellar clinical career and positive beginnings in early leadership positions may begin to fall short of what is needed to succeed at the highest levels of the organization. Executive failure is commonplace, but the research suggests that derailment can be caught and, if detected early enough, corrected.

> Hiring the wrong VPMA cost our organization far more than I can ever imagine.
> —*Anonymous CEO, 2012*

This issue is alarming for physician leadership. Consider the following: "Leadership derailment is unfortunately quite pervasive, with a 47 percent failure rate of management and leaders" (Hogan, Hogan, and Kaiser 2011).

Given the research support, considering and trying to better understand the risk of derailment will prove to be an important investment.

CAUSES

Research suggests that the following are the key reasons for derailment:

- Lack of a flexible leadership style
- Problems with interpersonal relationships
- Not meeting objectives
- Failure to lead a team
- Inability to adapt during a transition

These reasons have special significance for physicians.

Flexible leadership style. Physicians have usually worked in clinical settings where their authority is final (the buck stops with them). They seldom have had the chance to work collaboratively; their developed style results from being ultimately responsible for care of the patient.

Interpersonal relationships. Many physicians come from clinical experiences where they are not challenged and they do not learn the requisite skills of persuasion, listening, and empathy, all skills required of strong leaders. Even though physicians may have excellent interpersonal skills ("bedside manner") with their patients, this often does not translate to the management conference room.

Failure to meet objectives. Unfortunately, many physician leadership positions have few quantitative objectives; the task at hand is often laden with the subjectivity of human interaction. Physician executives are often evaluated solely on how they persuade, flatter, and direct the activities of others.

Failure to lead a team. Although more contemporary medicine has started to use teams more in the clinical setting, most physician leaders have not hired team members, formed teams, and led teams. Most physician activity relating to the care of patients involves the scientific analysis of quantitative clinical measures (evidence-based practice); leading teams is more of an art and much less of a science.

Inability to adapt during a transition. The move from clinical practice to a management or leadership position is an enormous transition. The problem of the transition can be exacerbated when physicians, being individuals not accustomed to failing, underestimate the challenges of the transition. The ability to sell change, to get approval for projects or budgets, or to navigate the confusion of the typical organizational chart can create real challenges for the new physician executive.

Ignoring politics. Politics, good and bad, exist in every organization, and managing them is crucial. Often physicians fail to realize this factor fully because they have not been part of the typical organizational jockeying that occurs in a leadership environment. One of the issues that may cause political trouble is being overly ambitious, which is particularly an issue with physicians (see "Some Indications of Trouble"). Physicians typically are driven and competitive, which can lead to problems in leadership situations. Effective leaders need ambition to be successful; one mark of strong leadership is the drive to make things better. But individuals who are more competitive may also exhibit drive that is extreme. Dye and Garman (2006) explain that personal drive that gets out of control "can be detrimental [and can] allow personal goals to become the end-all, be-all *raison d'etre*." This can cause other common problems that often surface with physician leaders, such as lack of sensitivity to other people and failing to manage political issues effectively.

Some Indications of Trouble

Most nonphysician executives received coaching and mentoring during their 20s, practiced it in their 30s, and are already well honed by the time they reach their 40s. Many physicians, however, start their first leadership position in their 40s, which can be like an athlete playing in a world championship game without the prerequisite time in the minor leagues. Physicians have also been educated in a milieu that assumes that once they are trained (clinically at least), admitting anything less than total proficiency is a sign of weakness or even failure. This attitude can easily spill over into management and leadership. Therefore, organizations must watch for early signs of derailment. Your physician leaders may be headed for derailment if they make statements such as these:

- "I got here alone, and I don't need any help."
- "I cannot delegate. My work is too important."
- "I have always been a winner."
- "I was a great medical staff president, and I will be a great chief medical officer."
- "I am an admiral, and I will decide where the ship goes."
- "Leadership courses? Nope, not for me."
- "I really don't need help. I can do this."

One significant cause of derailment is caustic behavior at the interpersonal level. Because most physicians begin their first leadership positions as already seasoned individuals, it is assumed that they are skilled at interpersonal relationships. Yet this is often not the case. Carson and colleagues (2012) used the psychologist Karen Horney's coping theories to determine primary causes of derailment. Horney posited that when interpersonal problems arise, individuals manage those relationships in one of four ways—moving with (the only healthy approach of the four), moving against, moving toward, or moving away. Exhibit 15.1 describes the four coping mechanisms. Those who *move against* will use their power with others and are often sarcastic or distrustful. Those who *move away* are often indifferent or insensitive to others' feelings. Those who *move toward* have an intense need to be liked and will often try to please or defer to others. Finally, those who *move with* are healthy in their interpersonal relationships, get along well with others, and work well in teams.

Exhibit 15.1: Karen Horney's Coping Mechanisms

Psychological Behavior	Horney Label	Leader Derailer
Aggressive	Moving against	Dictatorial; domineering
Dependent	Moving toward	Unable to make decisions; analysis paralysis
Withdrawing	Moving away	Aloof; can do it all without a team
Healthy	Moving with	Positive leader—no derailers

SOURCE: Adapted from Horney (1937).

Carson and colleagues' study showed that most leaders who derailed tended to move against others. They concluded that it was the "qualities that rub up badly against others, such as attention-seeking, idiosyncrasy, over-confidence and rule-bending (that) translate into red-flag behaviors (and) that predict early exit from the organization."

Remedies for Derailment

Identify weaknesses and work on them. In the past ten years, a fad called *strength-based development* has suggested ignoring weaknesses and instead only emphasizing strengths. This popular theory of professional development unfortunately does not have any research to back its contention. Moreover, it is founded on "positive psychology," which tries to address the view of psychology as being only negative. The book *The Perils of Accentuating the Positive* (Kaiser 2009) offsets this trend and suggests that a firm understanding of weaknesses and a willingness to improve is a foundation for success. Physicians need to be told of managerial or leadership weaknesses and given suggestions for improvement.

Identify areas of stress or complexity and manage their effects. Derailment behaviors may surface because of stress. As physician leaders move into their positions, they often find that many of the issues they need to manage are very complex and have far-reaching political characteristics with no clear-cut resolutions. Also, when leaders are confronted by unique problems or strategic choices with no apparent choice, stress can result. Physician leaders should not be expected to be always able to handle these complexities.

Provide specific feedback on performance evaluations. The higher in an organization executives move, the less likely they are to receive feedback about their behavior. And yet, for many physician leaders, their success rests in great part on political and interpersonal skills. In the words of a number of leadership experts, leaders are hired for past results and fired for personality. Executive performance evaluations often focus exclusively on organizational parameters of success—profitability, meeting budget, quality scores, and patient satisfaction scores—rather than personal factors. However, leaders sometimes have little influence over these factors and would benefit instead from specific insight on their people skills, such as communication, collaboration, and conflict management.

Identify strengths that can become weaknesses. A physician's strengths can often become her weaknesses. The bold and confident leader or manager can easily become arrogant and bigheaded. Creativity can turn into rule breaking. Even a sense of humor can upset progress in some negotiations. Sometimes this results from a leader being a "one-trick pony"—or, as one physician executive said, "If the only tool you have is a hammer, everything starts to look like a nail."

Watch for overconfidence. Although this remedy could easily fit under the prior heading, we present it separately because our experience has taught us that it can be one of the biggest derailers of physician leaders. In society and inside healthcare organizations, physicians hold a position of high esteem, and as such, they are often not challenged or corrected. This reverence often leads to overconfidence. Leaders often fall in love with their visions and strategies and fail to pull the plug soon enough, especially when others are hesitant to question or challenge them. Self-confidence is also sometimes inversely related to self-perception—it may block the ability to reflect and assess oneself more objectively.

Manage the transition formally and carefully. Morgan McCall (1998), one of the early researchers on derailment, indicated the demands involved in making a transition can cause derailment. The transition from being a clinician to being a leader or manager carries the same type of risks.

Physician to Physician

To avoid derailment, physician executives—indeed, all physician leaders—must know precisely their strengths and weaknesses.
—Jacque Sokolov, MD

GETTING HELP

Organizations should protect themselves against possible derailment of their physician leaders. Implementing an exceptional assessment and selection process (as discussed in Chapter 12) is the first step. Putting into operation a highly effective on-boarding and orientation program will be helpful as well. Some new physician leaders may need special support. Enrolling some in a formal master's degree program may be useful, while others may benefit from a formal coaching or mentoring program. Some organizations have found it useful to help the new physician leader connect with two or three other new physician leaders. Networking with leaders in other organizations can create a great support system. Organizations such as The Healthcare Roundtable provide the small support group atmosphere that allows new executives to develop helpful relationships.

Perhaps more important than the tools and processes is the commitment of executives to dedicate time to engaging their newly selected physician leaders in discussions about their challenges and solutions. Just having a more seasoned executive who is comfortable and savvy enough to challenge the physician leader without being intimidated can be helpful.

On a personal basis, physician managers and executives would do well to be vigilant about recognizing the signals of early derailment and to surround themselves with help. Assistance can come in several forms.

Get feedback about performance. Many leaders have a handful of individuals on whom they rely to give them feedback about organizational issues. Many physician executives regularly drop in on the medical staff lounge or eat in the doctors' dining room to see how things are going. While this effort is admirable, it may not provide statistically significant inputs. Physicians should know that a representative sampling increases the probability that an observation is correct. So, using more formal methods to collect input data on performance may be necessary. One of the best vehicles is a 360-degree evaluation tool that provides input from subordinates, peers, and superiors. Tools can be developed around specific job behaviors, leadership competencies, and perceptions of effectiveness and results.

Consider executive coaching. Executive coaching is a good service for a physician executive. Some newly hired physician leaders insist that they be provided some coaching. Keep in mind that executive coaching is not designed only for those executives who are in trouble; in fact, contemporary executive coaching is focused on individual growth related specifically to the job and its role and objectives. Effective executive coaches do not primarily concentrate on the psychology of leadership unless it is related to the job. Good coaches understand the work environment, and most have been executives or have worked on leadership teams.

They understand the executive leadership process and organizational dynamics. And, although industrial psychologists with strong experience in the working world often provide effective coaching support, some believe that physician leaders clearly need coaching from other physician leaders because of the special nature of the guild environment.

Network. Joining networking groups can be helpful. Physicians, although independent, do come together in groups to learn. Physician executive networking groups can provide an opportunity to discuss best practices and discover new ways to approach issues and problems.

Be a lifelong learner. The most successful executives typically have the following characteristics:

◆ They are willing to learn new skills and to learn about effective leadership behaviors.
◆ They typically prepare themselves for physician management and leadership positions.
◆ They seek out continuing education.
◆ They are less self-centered on a personal basis and get along well with others.
◆ They are willing to admit mistakes and seek to learn from them. Openness is a common trait.

On-boarding is essential. An effective organizational on-boarding program can help ensure physician management and leadership success. Physicians who move into these roles are making significant career and life changes. This transition must be supplemented with steady support. New skills need to be developed and used, and an expert needs to guide this process. Feedback must be given (and accepted). Use this time to have frank discussion of how some of the skills and strengths that served the physician well in a prior role might become liabilities.

On-boarding is a relatively new concept, and its practice varies greatly from organization to organization. The authors strongly feel that the most effective on-boarding programs are guided by an outside expert. Some situations may require that a neutral outsider guide the process because no matter how skilled internal people may be, they will have personal allegiances and loyalties to others on the inside. Giving the newly hired physician an impartial and nonaligned guide may be the best investment an organization can make.

Use formal evaluation systems. Formal evaluations can be helpful if they are competency-based and provide behavioral examples so physicians can identify the areas of concern. Generic descriptors are of little use, particularly to physicians, who think much more scientifically. If early signs of misstep occur, the annual

Exhibit 15.2: Listening Problem Areas and Solutions

Possible Problem Area	Solution
Trying to solve the problem described	Consider turning the tables and asking for a suggested solution.
Allowing distractions to cloud what is heard	Set aside a specific physical location for listening and remove phones, Blackberries, and other distractions.
Not allowing adequate time for the presentation of an issue or problem	Ask the person to return at a better time, ask for a written statement of the issue and suggested solutions, or ask for more time to study the issue.
Missing nonverbal cues or the deeper meaning of the message	Ask for clarification by restating the concern or issue or by stating, "I do not know what you mean."
Lacking empathy or failing to identify with the communicator or the message	State the obvious—that you are genuinely concerned.
Believing you have "been there and done that," and you already know the solution	Don't interrupt; allow the full message to be presented.
Dealing with a hot and emotional topic	Stay calm and clear-headed; learn that some matters can be put off until tomorrow.

evaluation system may catch problems too late. To avoid this issue, organizations would be wise to conduct evaluations on a more frequent basis with newer physician executives.

Create a "no blame" culture. In 1999, the Institute of Medicine (IOM) released its report *To Err Is Human: Building a Safer Health System* and introduced the concept of a "no blame" culture, which enhances patient safety by shifting the blame for mistakes from the individual to the environment. Organizations also must develop leadership cultures that do not seek to assign blame when problems occur. Supportive growth and development in an environment that embraces diverse thought and creativity means that mistakes will be made.

Listening. New physician leaders must hone their listening skills. After several years of clinical practice, where the bulk of the listening was done almost exclusively with patients, physicians may find the need to raise their level of focus in this area. Exhibit 15.2 provides several simple but powerful listening suggestions.

CONCLUSION

We close this chapter with a simple word: "Beware." Do not avoid careful consideration of the threat of derailment. The costs both to the physician who must make a life change and to the organization are immense.

Thoughts for Consideration

Do you have feedback mechanisms to catch early problems that might cause later derailments?

Does the daily pressure and busyness of the job interfere with the need to capture information about performance?

Has your organization's leadership development program delved into the topic of managerial derailment?

Do you provide executive coaching to new physician leaders?

SUGGESTED READING

Furnham, A. 2010. *The Elephant in the Boardroom: The Causes of Leadership Derailment.* Basingstoke, UK: Palgrave Macmillan.

Gentry, W. A., S. P. Mondore, and B. D. Cox. 2007. "A Study of Managerial Derailment Characteristics and Personality Preferences." *Journal of Management Development* 26 (9): 857–73.

Hogan, J., R. Hogan, and R. B. Kaiser. 2011. "Management Derailment." In *American Psychological Association Handbook of Industrial and Organizational Psychology.* Washington, DC: American Psychological Association.

Patterson, K., J. Grenny, R. McMillan, and A. Switzler. 2002. *Crucial Conversations: Tools for Talking When Stakes Are High.* New York: McGraw-Hill.

A Note from the Authors

A great deal has changed since we started writing this book. The results of the national election are in, and "Obamacare" (the Patient Protection and Affordable Care Act of 2010) is clearly going to have significant influence in the industry for the next several years. Moreover, the reform law passed Supreme Court muster in late June 2012 and many organizations in the healthcare industry have already made major changes in their strategy, including forming accountable care organizations (ACOs) and clinically integrated organizations (CIOs), building collaborative relationships, and looking at further ways to join forces.

Much consolidation has taken place among Catholic healthcare organizations and in academic medical centers, and more is likely to come. The scale of many of the consolidations suggests that extremely large systems will be created in the next few years. Some new collaborations provide significant geographic diversification and "virtual" mergers. Even smaller organizations that have vowed to remain independent for years are now considering significant partnering arrangements. Moreover, the federal Medicare program and the state Medicaid programs clearly will have to make substantial cuts in reimbursement. Hospitals and health systems are taking critical looks at organizational transformation and other tactics to address the challenges. And the quality improvement movement continues to grow. These events add considerable clarity to the shape of the healthcare market and the place that value-based purchasing arrangements and better focused, better coordinated patient care—clinical integration, in other words—will have in tomorrow's healthcare system. The election results, the Supreme Court ruling, and the other changes did not, of course, have a huge impact on the need for physician leadership; the need already existed. But as these changes and transformations of our industry occur, additional physician involvement and leadership will be crucial.

The fact is nothing will slow the development of CIOs and the need to participate in multiple value-based products. The complexity of implementing CIOs from a regulatory standpoint remains and requires a significant level of expertise to execute properly. The clinical model that affects integration and physician leadership will continue to evolve on the following fronts:

1. What exists within a CIO today needs to be optimized; in other words, we need to keep doing what we do today, only better.
2. From an enterprise clinical model consideration, the medical staff must continue to be involved in more discussions.
3. The existing clinical model will continue to be transformed into one with fewer physicians and more collaborative care methodologies. All of those are evolving and will continue to do so in the intermediate to long-term time frame.
4. As larger organizations are formed, physician leadership will be required to lead the transformation.

Of course, clinical integration exists in *local* healthcare markets, and markets in general have had a varied evolution in the expense, speed, and development of CIOs. The primary variables are whether a value-based commercial product or a large ACO development effort has been introduced in a given market and how many organizations in a local market have started to form ACOs or CIOs, whether or not any insurance-driven systems have been developed, and the extent to which large providers get into the insurance market. Either of the two value-based products—one for the commercial market and one for Medicare—can cause other CIOs to form and produce value-based products to compete against other delivery systems. With the 2014 health insurance exchanges imminent, initiatives to build CIOs capable of offering a value-based product are only going to accelerate.

And looking even further down the road, we see the concept of population health, which to us means a healthcare organization taking responsibility for the health outcomes of a group of individuals and the practices that impact their health and wellness. We feel confident that physicians, often armed with additional training in public health and epidemiology, will help lead organizations as they deal not only with healthcare but also with public health education, prevention and interventions, physical and social environmental issues, the impact of genetics on health and wellness, and coaching individuals to engage in healthy behavior. CIOs will require physicians who have considerable understanding of population health and its management. This will prompt further demand for physician leadership and involvement.

But regardless of the local market, regulations drive the form of organizations that will deliver care, the manner in which all this work is paid for, and the management of population health. The real issue of the future is how physicians will increasingly be involved as active participants and as assertive leaders in these endeavors. For too long, physicians have been on the sidelines of many healthcare organizations, and while they have been actively caring for patients and providing clinical services, they have not been major drivers of strategy and change. Those days must end if clinical integration is fully developed—the imperatives of the future require much more active physician involvement and leadership.

An Institute of Medicine (2012) study describes our healthcare system as being too complex and costly to continue business as usual. The report focuses on inefficiencies, an inability to manage a rapidly deepening clinical knowledge base, and a reward system poorly focused on patient needs. Clearly, turning the system around will require expert physician leadership.

In closing, healthcare reform, cost cutting, care shifting to different locations, CIOs, enhanced quality and patient safety, team-based patient care, clinical transformation, value-based payment for care, population health—these all begin and end with physician leadership. Colmers (2011) writes that "the Reform River is a raging torrent." Truly the changes ahead are massive and only the best-led organizations will thrive. We hope we have made a compelling argument to increase and enhance physician leadership and involvement in the strategy development and operations management of the healthcare organization. Some may not perceive that there is any burning platform to do so, and others will say they have already done enough with physician leadership development. In our view, only the surface has been scratched, and the efforts must go much further. We urge serious consideration of our premises. We believe the future of our healthcare delivery system depends on it.

Good luck.

—*Carson and Jacque*
November 2012

Evaluation Tool—Physician Leadership and Involvement Program

This tool is not intended to cover all aspects of physician leadership, but it provides a good starting point for leaders to evaluate their efforts toward the creation of a physician leadership development program.

The questions could be used as discussion guides with groups of physician leaders and nonphysician leaders. These could be used as the framework for a strategic planning retreat or a series of meetings over time where the intent is to build a strategic and tactical plan to address physician leadership development.

IDENTIFYING YOUR PHYSICIAN LEADERS

Please answer the following questions (truthfully):

1. Have you identified physician leaders in your organization?
2. Has this identification process been formal?
3. Do those who have been identified know they have been identified?
4. How did you identify them?
   List specific criteria you used in identifying physician leaders:
   a.
   b.
   c.
   d.
   e.
   f.
   g.

h.

i.

5. (For nonphysicians in the group) When identifying physician leaders, did you get any input from other physicians in the identification process (either formally or informally)?

6. Are the identified leaders part of the formal medical staff leadership group? Employed physician group?

7. Is your formal leadership composed of elected leaders or employed physicians, or some combination of both?

Can you point to specific tools and practices that indicate that physician leadership selection is based on any of the following?

1. Identify and select based on specific leadership competencies and experience.
2. Identify and select based on interest/aspiration level.
3. Identify representation from all areas of the medical staff, with special emphasis on primary care (or some other area).
4. Identify and select based on knowledge of process improvement (Lean, Six Sigma, continuous quality improvement).
5. Identify and select based on interest in utilization review, operation issues, and understanding of cost containment.
6. Identify and select based on working knowledge of insurance and managed care.
7. Identify and select based on willingness to be coached and mentored.
8. Identify and select based on communication skills, both written and verbal.
9. Identify and select based on history as excellent clinician. While there is usually not time or the need for the physician executive to practice medicine, the individual must have a reputation as a solid practitioner to have credibility with the medical staff. This is true for both the internal and external candidate.
10. Identify and select based on negotiating skills.
11. Identify and select based on vision/strategic planning skills and knowledge.
12. Identify and select based on diplomacy and tact.
13. Identify and select based on a desire to be part of the healthcare solution.
14. Identify and select based on ability as a risk-taker.
15. Identify and select based on the fit with the culture and the mission of the organization.

PHYSICIAN COMMUNICATIONS

Is your communications program with your physicians addressing some or all of the following?

- Monitoring the effectiveness of efforts to communicate with physicians is ongoing.
- Successful communication plans are reflected by long-term commitment to being transparent and open.
- Commitment to providing information and opportunity for input must come from senior leaders.
- All staff members believe in the commitment to communicating with physicians.
- An organizational comfort level exists in communicating with physicians.
- There is no us-versus-them mentality.
- There is a comprehensive communications plan.
- The organization does not rely on only one form of communication.
- The organization uses emerging social media and other newer generation modalities.
- The organization understands that the medical staff is not homogenous.
- The organization places *more* emphasis on:
  - Personal meetings
  - Task force and advisory board involvement
  - Using credible messengers
  - Building rapport and credibility with all physician groups
  - Respect for time—effective meeting management and true need for meetings
  - Communications with those physicians who do not come to the acute care hospital as much
- And places *less* emphasis on:
  - Letters and phone calls
  - Newsletters
  - Visits to physicians only from physician services representatives
  - Bulletin board messages
  - Just showing up in the medical staff lounge

CURRICULUM IN PROGRAMS

The organization has carefully thought through the curriculum and has addressed at least the following:

1. Program is targeted at multiple audiences:
   - Unpaid (volunteer) administrative physicians
   - Part-time and full-time paid physician leaders
   - Physicians who are full-time clinicians but are "leaders" or exhibit leadership tendencies
   - Those who are in management positions and those who are in leadership positions
2. Program provides:
   A. Leadership thought and theory
   B. Strategic management of an enterprise
   C. Principles of management
   D. Group process
   E. Change management
   F. Conflict management
   G. Negotiations
   H. Legal aspects
   I. Current trends in healthcare delivery and financing
   J. Skill building
   K. Meeting management
3. Program is developed around the following tracks:
   A. Introduction to leadership
   B. Financial management
   C. Organizational management
   D. Strategy
4. Curriculum is:
   A. Coordinated
   B. Structured on an annual basis
   C. Incremental
5. Program is built around real case studies.
6. Program also provides significant opportunity to experientially apply what is learned.

ADDITIONAL CONSIDERATIONS

1. Do multiple physicians regularly interact with members of senior management?
    - Yes, frequently
    - Yes, occasionally
    - Infrequently
    - Not at all
2. Have physicians (other than the VPMA) ever attended a regular meeting of the senior management?
    - Yes
    - No
3. The quality of input from physicians into senior management decisions is:

Very Unsatisfactory	Unsatisfactory	Neither Satisfactory nor Unsatisfactory	Satisfactory	Very Satisfactory
1	2	3	4	5

4. The quantity of input from physicians into senior management decisions is:

Very Unsatisfactory	Unsatisfactory	Neither Satisfactory nor Unsatisfactory	Satisfactory	Very Satisfactory
1	2	3	4	5

5. Has a physician (other than the VPMA) given a presentation at a *routine* senior management meeting?
    - Yes
    - No
6. Do physicians attend any regular meetings of the middle management team?
    - Yes
    - No
7. Has a physician (other than the VPMA) given a presentation at a *routine* middle management meeting?
    - Yes
    - No

8. Are physicians part of the budget process?
   - Yes
   - Somewhat
   - No
9. The *degree* of involvement of physicians in the budget process is:

Very Unsatisfactory	Unsatisfactory	Neither Satisfactory nor Unsatisfactory	Satisfactory	Very Satisfactory
1	2	3	4	5

10. The quality and quantity of the input (consider the degree of appropriate influence) by physicians into the budget process is:

Very Unsatisfactory	Unsatisfactory	Neither Satisfactory nor Unsatisfactory	Satisfactory	Very Satisfactory
1	2	3	4	5

11. The quality of involvement of physicians in the formal process of strategic planning is positive.

Strongly Disagree	Disagree	Neither Disagree nor Agree	Agree	Strongly Agree
1	2	3	4	5

12. The quantity of involvement of physicians in the formal process of strategic planning is positive.

Strongly Disagree	Disagree	Neither Disagree nor Agree	Agree	Strongly Agree
1	2	3	4	5

13. One of the topic headings of the organization's strategic plan relates to physician involvement.

Strongly Disagree	Disagree	Neither Disagree nor Agree	Agree	Strongly Agree
1	2	3	4	5

14. One of the topic headings of the organization's strategic plan relates to physician leadership.

Strongly Disagree	Disagree	Neither Disagree nor Agree	Agree	Strongly Agree
1	2	3	4	5

15. Physicians play a regular part in the ongoing adjustments and modifications to the organization's strategic plan.

Strongly Disagree	Disagree	Neither Disagree nor Agree	Agree	Strongly Agree
1	2	3	4	5

16. Physician leaders understand the process of strategic planning.

Strongly Disagree	Disagree	Neither Disagree nor Agree	Agree	Strongly Agree
1	2	3	4	5

17. The timing and pace of change involved in strategic initiatives is appropriate for the physician community of the organization.

Strongly Disagree	Disagree	Neither Disagree nor Agree	Agree	Strongly Agree
1	2	3	4	5

18. The development of the vision for the future of the organization is done concurrently with the involvement of the physician leaders of the organization.

Strongly Disagree	Disagree	Neither Disagree nor Agree	Agree	Strongly Agree
1	2	3	4	5

19. The medical staff organization is appropriately involved and organized to support and energize the physician group to overcome political and bureaucratic barriers to change.

Strongly Disagree	Disagree	Neither Disagree nor Agree	Agree	Strongly Agree
1	2	3	4	5

20. The organization's strategic focus can best be described as physician driven.

Strongly Disagree	Disagree	Neither Disagree nor Agree	Agree	Strongly Agree
1	2	3	4	5

21. The general medical staff is knowledgeable of and supports the strategic plan of the organization.

Strongly Disagree	Disagree	Neither Disagree nor Agree	Agree	Strongly Agree
1	2	3	4	5

22. As one of the key components of the development of the strategic plan, the entire medical staff is involved.

Strongly Disagree	Disagree	Neither Disagree nor Agree	Agree	Strongly Agree
1	2	3	4	5

23. Informal physician leaders (unpaid but influential) would describe decisions made by the organization by using the pronoun and verb "we decided."

Strongly Disagree	Disagree	Neither Disagree nor Agree	Agree	Strongly Agree
1	2	3	4	5

24. Additional attention is focused on building and maintaining relationships with those physicians who are not closely tied to the organization (e.g., physicians in remote office locations).

Strongly Disagree	Disagree	Neither Disagree nor Agree	Agree	Strongly Agree
1	2	3	4	5

25. Leadership of the organization is sensitive to the pace of change of factors that impact physician activity.

Strongly Disagree	Disagree	Neither Disagree nor Agree	Agree	Strongly Agree
1	2	3	4	5

26. Physician leadership is integrally involved as a "steering" decision maker in information systems strategies and initiatives.

Strongly Disagree	Disagree	Neither Disagree nor Agree	Agree	Strongly Agree
1	2	3	4	5

27. A strong positive feeling exists about physician contributions to the overall success of the organization.

Strongly Disagree	Disagree	Neither Disagree nor Agree	Agree	Strongly Agree
1	2	3	4	5

28. Patient decisions are physician driven.

Strongly Disagree	Disagree	Neither Disagree nor Agree	Agree	Strongly Agree
1	2	3	4	5

29. Physicians would defend the status and reputation of the organization if it were attacked.

Strongly Disagree	Disagree	Neither Disagree nor Agree	Agree	Strongly Agree
1	2	3	4	5

30. Physicians would indicate they have a lot of personal say-so and control in organizational decision making.

Strongly Disagree	Disagree	Neither Disagree nor Agree	Agree	Strongly Agree
1	2	3	4	5

31. Physicians would describe the organization as "their" organization.

Strongly Disagree	Disagree	Neither Disagree nor Agree	Agree	Strongly Agree
1	2	3	4	5

Clinical Integration Readiness Assessment

ARE YOU READY?

Clinical integration isn't an approach to healthcare delivery and reimbursement that you decide to pursue one day and put in place the next. Your institution needs to be ready for it, and that readiness crosses departments, facilities, and provider organizations. To assess your readiness for clinical integration, determine where you are on this roadmap—and whether you can realistically follow it to its end.

Fast-Track Start

0–3 Months

- Physicians largely resistant to change
- Limited physician–hospital collaboration
- Traditional medical directorships, but no real team-based care or comanagement of clinical services

3–6 Months

- Several service-line comanagement arrangements in place
- Physician-centric hospital-sponsored medical group structure functioning
- Joint physician–hospital planning committee in place

6–12 Months

- Additional service-line comanagement arrangements crafted
- Pluralistic physician–hospital governance structure in place
- Task force to start work on the design of the ultimate CIO

12–18 Months

- The CIO is fully operational, but the clinical model continues to evolve
- Initial VBP payer contracts are being negotiated

18 Months and Beyond

- Ability to deliver superior performance; quality/cost quantitative metrics in place
- Capable of managing full risk for a population or product

That is the overview. The specific questions you need to ask yourself to determine if you're prepared to move to meaningful clinical integration include the following:

- Do you have a provider-sponsored integrated network in place?
- Does that network meet federal meaningful clinical integration requirements?
- Are you ready to plug into a variety of value-based purchasing (VBP) products with a variety of payers? That includes Medicare, Medicaid, health insurance exchanges, commercial plans, regional networks, and super CIOs.
- Do you have attractive geographic coverage?
- Are you the network of choice in your market?
- Here is the holy grail of clinical integration readiness on the way to VBP: Are you an indispensable provider in your market?
- Are you capable of superior performance? That includes quality, patient safety, appropriate resource utilization, and patient and provider satisfaction.
- Do you have a proven ability to manage risk effectively?
- Can your organization meet the Federal Trade Commission's checklist for meaningful clinical integration?
  - Can you show clear integration and interdependence among providers?
  - Do you have in-network referrals of both primary and specialty physicians in place?
  - Do you have development, training, promotion, and tracking of clinical standards, benchmarks, and protocols in place?

- – Do you have an integrated IT platform? That means both efficient exchange of clinical information across the care continuum and utilization data gathered, analyzed, and shared with CIO providers.
  - – Do you have defined processes for tracking provider adherence to protocols?
- ◆ More generally, do you have a network scaled to deliver care across all settings and specialties?
- ◆ Do you have a legal framework and capabilities to enable joint contracting and single-signature authority?
- ◆ Do you have a well-defined governance and decision-making structure?
- ◆ Is there clear alignment of financial incentives among participants toward common objectives?
- ◆ Are you capable of accepting common financial risk for performance and of internally distributing revenues and expenses?
- ◆ Do you have sufficient numbers of patients to support comprehensive performance measurement and reporting?
- ◆ Are physicians engaged with you in trying to accomplish strategic goals? That includes such important areas as clinical program growth, management of cost and quality, integration and collaboration, and adoption of electronic medical records and connectivity tools.
- ◆ Are physicians involved in clinical program management?
- ◆ Are you partnering with physicians economically?
- ◆ Do you have an effective physician–hospital governance or management model?
- ◆ Are payers in your market developing VBP agreements?
- ◆ What is the general consensus among payers regarding contracting with provider-developed CIO or super CIO networks?
- ◆ Are your competitors developing CIOs or super CIOs?
- ◆ Are they purchasing practices and employing physicians?
- ◆ Are they pursuing strategies for growing market share?
- ◆ What are the key trends in your market?
- ◆ What is the existing balance of power between payers and providers?
- ◆ What is the potential for hospital consolidation? Who will likely be the dominant players?

Now you know where you stand. Are you ready?

Letters

LETTERS TO PHYSICIANS WHO HAVE EXPRESSED INTEREST IN LEADERSHIP OPPORTUNITIES

Much of our book has focused on how physicians can transition into management and leadership positions and how they can best be prepared for success in those roles. The following sample letters are not necessarily meant to be used as actual letters. Instead, they provide guidance on the areas of focus that are helpful to physicians who have realized they would like to step into a different role. The first letter is addressed to those physicians who do not plan to leave clinical practice entirely but want to engage in some leadership activity on a part-time basis. The second letter is addressed to physicians wanting to move full-time into leadership and leave clinical practice.

LETTER TO PHYSICIAN WHO WANTS TO ADD LEADERSHIP OPPORTUNITIES TO A CLINICAL PRACTICE

Dear Dr. [NAME]:

You have expressed an interest in adding valuable leadership responsibilities on top of your extremely important clinical practice here at [INSTITUTION NAME]. Thank you very much for your interest!

We have learned from experience that taking two very important next steps will help ensure that your expectations for maximizing your leadership opportunities match our needs, and that both parties, you and [INSTITUTION], get the most out of our continuing collaboration. You will see details in the attached appendix.

To start, we recommend "buffing and polishing" your clinical core competencies so that you can bring clinical excellence to whatever leadership position you eventually fill. In addition, we recommend making a careful determination of where you want to be a part of [INSTITUTION NAME]'s leadership—at the governance, management, or operations level. Making that decision will help you focus your educational efforts to prepare yourself for a leadership position with us.

We look forward to working together as you continue to pursue career opportunities at [INSTITUTION]. Thank you very much!

[SIGNATURE OF HOSPITAL EXECUTIVE]

Appendix to Letter

Step One: Shore up your clinical core competencies.

Make absolutely sure that your clinical skills foundation is as developed as it can be. Are all of your certifications up-to-date, for example? Have you completed all appropriate and relevant clinical coursework? Making sure your qualifications are a foundation of strong clinical excellence will help ensure maximum credibility in the areas of leadership you want to pursue.

Step Two: Identify whether your leadership goals are primarily in governance, management, or operations.

- If you are primarily interested in governance opportunities, educating yourself on the fundamentals of governance—such as the structure, function, and responsibilities of a board of directors—will help.
- If you want to go into management, you will need to be clear about what you want to manage. Are you interested in management at the enterprise level, such as a CEO position? Are you more interested in a specific area of responsibility, such as a vice president of medical affairs position or a chief quality officer position? Start by developing a focused approach to general management skills—for example, by earning a master's in business administration—then focus on your specific management skill and what you are trying to achieve.

- If you are interested in a leadership role in operations, which usually involves clinical operations, start now to develop relationships within your area of expertise, such as finance, enterprisewide operations, or perhaps a clinical service line, to take on specific operations responsibilities—such as through a mentorship or apprenticeship opportunity—to develop your operations skill set.

LETTER TO PHYSICIAN WHO WANTS TO MOVE INTO LEADERSHIP OPPORTUNITIES AND LEAVE CLINICAL PRACTICE BEHIND

Dear Dr. [NAME]:

You have expressed an interest in moving from a primary focus on clinical practice here at [INSTITUTION NAME] into a full-time leadership position with us. Thank you very much for your interest!

We have learned from experience that taking four very important steps will help ensure that your expectations for maximizing your leadership opportunities match our needs and that both parties, you and [INSTITUTION], get the most out of our continuing collaboration. You'll see details in the attached appendix.

First, we recommend that you determine what area of leadership you want to make your new career pathway. We have learned from experience that for a physician to make a living by simply serving on a board of directors is rare, unless you plan to retire and you are separately financially secure. Second, we recommend that you "buff and polish" your clinical core competencies so that you can bring clinical excellence to whatever leadership position you eventually fill.

Third, we recommend making a careful determination of where you want to be a part of [INSTITUTION NAME]— at the governance, management, or operations level. That decision will help you focus your educational efforts to prepare yourself for a leadership position with us. And finally, we recommend that you determine the best time to make your move, and whether it involves phasing out your clinical practice or an all-or-nothing strategy of moving directly into a full-time leadership position.

We look forward to working together as you continue to pursue your career opportunities at [INSTITUTION]. Thank you very much!

[SIGNATURE OF HOSPITAL EXECUTIVE]

Appendix to Letter

Step One: Determine, through a detailed exploratory process, your specific area of leadership interest.

An important exploratory process must occur regarding the skill sets and core competencies that you have versus those that you will need for the full-time leadership opportunities you want to move into. Also, you should decide what areas of healthcare you want to be a leader in:

◆ The payer side?
◆ The delivery system side?
◆ A physician organization?
◆ A hospital organization?
◆ Pharmacy?
◆ Medical devices?
◆ Information technology?

Are you interested in becoming a physician entrepreneur and creating a business that does not already exist? Or are you perhaps going to use insights or expertise you already have to develop a new or improved business and create a position for yourself in one of those areas? Visiting with individuals who have made the transition and shadowing them to better understand their jobs may be helpful.

Step Two: Be absolutely sure that your clinical skills foundation is as developed as it can be.

Are all of your certifications up-to-date? Have you completed all appropriate and relevant clinical coursework? Be sure that your qualifications are a foundation of strong clinical excellence; that will help ensure maximum credibility in the areas of leadership you want to pursue. This credibility will be helpful as you begin the new role; later, you will be judged more on your management and leadership skills and accomplishments.

Step Three: Identify whether your leadership goals are primarily in governance, management, or operations.

- If you are primarily interested in governance opportunities, educating yourself on the fundamentals of governance—such as the structure, function, and responsibilities of a board of directors—will help.
- If want to go into management, you will need to be clear about what you want to manage. Are you interested in management at the executive level, such as an operations or COO position? Are you more interested in a specific area of responsibility, such as a vice president of medical affairs position or a chief quality officer position? Start by developing a focused approach to general management skills—for example, by earning a master's in business administration—then focus on your specific management skill and what you are trying to achieve.
- If you are interested in a leadership role in operations, which usually involves clinical operations, start now to develop relationships within your area of expertise, such as finance, enterprisewide operations, or perhaps a clinical service line, to take on specific operations responsibilities—such as through a mentorship or apprenticeship opportunity—to develop your operations skill set.

Step Four: Determine the optimal timing for your planned career change.

Do you plan to phase out of clinical practice and into a leadership position? Do you plan to stop practicing and first pursue full-time a management-related degree, such as an MBA? We have found that the most common route to full-time leadership starts by looking at opportunities that present themselves for perhaps 20 to 30 percent of your time, then deciding based on real experience whether you want to pursue leadership full-time.

Physician Candidate Evaluations

SAMPLE I

This form is designed only as a sample start. Organizations are advised to customize forms to best fit their specific circumstances and position needs.

Sample
Senior Vice President of Medical Affairs
Candidate Evaluation Form

Candidate's Name: _____

Interviewer: _____

Candidates need to be evaluated and assessed based on their *specific past behaviors*. The principle of behavioral interviewing requires that candidates provide specific examples of how they have demonstrated specific skills and competencies in past jobs or situations. As you evaluate your interviewee, be certain that you have received specific examples that give you the ability to accurately assess the skills and competencies of the candidate. Please rate the candidate using the following scale: (circle choice) 1 – Low, 5 – High.

STRATEGIC SKILLS

	Low			High	
Developing specific strategies	1	2	3	4	5
Intellectual horsepower	1	2	3	4	5
Problem solving	1	2	3	4	5
Creativity	1	2	3	4	5
Broad strategic perspective	1	2	3	4	5

OPERATING TECHNICAL SKILLS

Financial management	1	2	3	4	5
Quality improvement skills	1	2	3	4	5
Team leadership skills	1	2	3	4	5
Board interaction skills	1	2	3	4	5

LEADERSHIP COMPETENCIES

Leadership/executive presence	1	2	3	4	5
Command skills	1	2	3	4	5
Conflict management	1	2	3	4	5
Physician relations	1	2	3	4	5
Making tough people calls	1	2	3	4	5
Hiring and staffing/reading people	1	2	3	4	5
Team player	1	2	3	4	5

ORGANIZATIONAL POSITIONING SKILLS

Organizational savvy	1	2	3	4	5
Organizational agility/flexibility	1	2	3	4	5
Political savvy	1	2	3	4	5
Communicating effectively	1	2	3	4	5
Presentation skills	1	2	3	4	5

INTERPERSONAL SKILLS

	Low			High	
Approachability	1	2	3	4	5
Interpersonal savvy	1	2	3	4	5
Caring about others	1	2	3	4	5
Compassion	1	2	3	4	5
Boss relationships	1	2	3	4	5
Customer focus	1	2	3	4	5
Ethics and values	1	2	3	4	5
Integrity and trust	1	2	3	4	5
Listening	1	2	3	4	5

FIT WITHIN SYSTEM

Prior system experience	1	2	3	4	5
Comfort with matrix relations	1	2	3	4	5
Team player within a system	1	2	3	4	5

OVERALL EVALUATION

1 2 3 4 5

Comments: _____

_____

_____

_____

_____

SAMPLE II

Interview Evaluation Form
Senior Vice President of Medical Affairs/Chief Quality Officer

The following criteria were developed to screen our SrVPMA/CQO candidates. Following your interview with each candidate, please rate the candidate against each of the criteria. If you are uncertain of their qualifications in any criteria, please mark it "NE" for "not evaluated." Please evaluate based on a five-point scale, five ("5") being the highest rating and one ("1") being the lowest rating.

+ Has a thorough knowledge of legal and regulatory requirements for physician integration/practice management. *Evaluation Score* _____
+ Has significant and progressive management experience and has demonstrated effectiveness in a large healthcare organization (experience as a VPMA, chief medical officer, chief quality officer, medical director, or the equivalent). *Evaluation Score* _____
+ Has knowledge and experience with quality infrastructure, including how to develop and implement decision tools, clinical protocols and guidelines, care management programs, and outcome measurement assessments. *Evaluation Score* _____
+ Has working knowledge of inpatient and outpatient clinical practice. *Evaluation Score* _____
+ Possesses working knowledge of electronic health records and information technology, including statistical analysis, clinical epidemiology, and medical informatics. Has a track record of leading clinical and performance improvement initiatives. *Evaluation Score* _____
+ Has extensive knowledge of national trends in quality with a history of collaboration in working with organizations, such as The Institute of Healthcare Improvement, National Quality Forum, The Joint Commission, and others. *Evaluation Score* _____
+ Has a philosophy of collaboration and teamwork and a demonstrable track record in forging physician/management relations. *Evaluation Score* _____
+ Has clinical credibility with physician constituencies. *Evaluation Score* _____
+ Has a high tolerance for complex, ambiguous, and ever-shifting environments, including a matrix management structure. *Evaluation Score* _____

- Possesses excellent interpersonal and communication skills, with a high premium given to the ability to build consensus; noticeable skills in engaging physicians and finding synergies; and an interactive style that is pleasant. ***Evaluation Score*** _____
- Is comfortable working in groups, forming teams of physicians and management, and working with other diverse collaborators. ***Evaluation Score*** _____
- Understands how to create change through influence and not through direct authority. ***Evaluation Score*** _____
- Is analytical, with the ability to draw conclusions from the data. Has expert knowledge of clinical effectiveness tools, including statistical analysis, epidemiology, continuous quality improvement, best practices, evidence-based medicine, and information technology. ***Evaluation Score*** _____
- Appreciates the importance of the clinical team, what nursing and operations bring to the patient care endeavor, and the strength of that clinical partnership. ***Evaluation Score*** _____
- Is able to be an appropriate advocate for the medical staff vantage point in promoting collaboration with administration and the board of trustees. ***Evaluation Score*** _____

Overall Rating (scale of 1 – 5, with 5 being the highest and 1 being the lowest):

_____ (Not an average of the above score but an overall impression)

References

The Advisory Board Company. 2012. "Building the Clinically Integrated Enterprise." Accessed October 15. www.advisory.com/Consulting/Southwind/Building-the-clinically-integrated-enterprise.

Advocate Health Care. 2012. "About Advocate Physician Partners." Accessed October 25. www.advocatehealth.com/app.

American Academy of Family Physicians (AAFP). 2012. "Patient-Centered Medical Home." Accessed November 5. www.aafp.org/online/en/home/policy/policies/p/patientcenteredmedhome.html.

American Medical Association (AMA). 2009. "Report of the Council on Ethical and Judicial Affairs: Physicians with Disruptive Behavior." Published March 1. www.ama-assn.org/ama1/pub/upload/mm/code-medical-ethics/ceja-3i09.pdf.

Anderson, D., B. Wieland, and R. Spiegel. 2011. "Clinical Integration: The Road to Accountable Care." Presented at Hospital and Physician Relations: An Executive Summit, October 19. www.bdcadvisors.com/uploads/October%202011%20The%20Road%20to%20Accountable%20Care,%20Hospital%20&%20Physician%20Relations%20Executive%20Summit.pdf.

Anderson, M. 2009. "How Do You Cope with Stress, Doctor?" *The Junior Doctor Blog.* Published March 4. http://thejuniordoctor.blogspot.com/2009/03/how-do-you-cope-with-stress-doctor.html.

Andrabi, I. 2012. "A Culture of Continuous Improvement Is Necessary for Success Under Value-Based Care." *Becker's Hospital Review.* Published February 23. www.beckershospitalreview.com/hospital-management-administration/a-culture-of-continuous-improvement-is-necessary-for-success-under-value-based-care.html.

Andrew, L. B. 1999. "Conflict Management, Prevention, and Resolution in Medical Settings." *The Physician Executive* 25 (4): 38–42.

Argyris, C. 1991. "Teaching Smart People How to Learn." *Harvard Business Review* 69 (3): 99–109.

Association of American Medical Colleges (AAMC). 2012. "AAMC Admissions Initiative." Accessed May 6. www.aamc.org/initiatives/admissions/.

———. 2005. *Recommendations for Clinical Skills Curricula for Undergraduate Medical Education.* Accessed May 6, 2012. https://members.aamc.org/eweb/DynamicPage.asp x?Activon=Add&ObjectKeyFrom=1A83491A-9853-4C87-86A4-F7D95601C2E2& WebCode=PubDetailAdd&DoNotSave=yes&ParentObject=CentralizedOrderEntry &ParentDataObject=Invoice%20Detail&ivd_formkey=69202792-63d7-4ba2-bf4e- a0da41270555&ivd_prc_prd_key=5E87BCBA-5AC9-4FA6-B64E-2F782AC59620.

Bakhtiari, E. 2008. "The Polarized Hospital–Physician Relationship." *HealthLeaders Media.* Published September 18. www.healthleadersmedia.com/content/PHY-219202/The-Polarized- HospitalPhysician-Relationship.html.

Blue Consulting Services. 2012. "Clinical Integration." Accessed October 15. http:// blueconsultingservices.com/physician-hospital-alignment/clinical-integration/.

Bogue, R. J., J. G. Guarneri, M. Reed, K. Bradley, and J. Hughes. 2006. "Secrets of Physician Satisfaction." *The Physician Executive* 32 (6): 30–39.

Bush, H. 2012. "Hospital Statistics Chart Rise in Physician Employment." *Hospitals and Health Networks Daily.* Published January 6. www.hhnmag.com/hhnmag/HHNDaily/ HHNDailyDisplay.dhtml?id=1970001363.

Carson, M. A., L. R. Shanock, E. D. Heggestad, A. M. Andrew, S. D. Pugh, and M. Walter. 2012. "The Relationship Between Dysfunctional Interpersonal Tendencies, Derailment Potential Behavior, and Turnover." *Journal of Business and Psychology* 27 (3): 291–304.

Center for Management Research. 2010. "Leadership Training and Development at P&G." Accessed June 12, 2012. www.icmrindia.org/casestudies/catalogue/Leadership%20and%20 Entrepreneurship/LDEN071.htm.

Centers for Medicare & Medicaid Services (CMS). 2007. "US Department of Health and Human Services Medicare Hospital Value-Based Purchasing Plan Development Issues Paper." Accessed October 29, 2012. www.cms.gov/Medicare/Medicare-Fee-for-Service-Payment/ AcuteInpatientPPS/Downloads/Hospital_VBP_Plan_Issues_Paper.pdf.

Churchill, W. 1952. Hansard, United Kingdom Parliament, Commons, HC Deb 04, volume 507, cc7-134. http://hansard.millbanksystems.com/commons/1952/nov/04/debate-on-the- address#S5CV0507P0_19521104_HOC_60.

Cohn, K., 2008. "Collaborative Mentality." *Healthcare Collaboration.* Published November 1. http://healthcarecollaboration.com/collaborative-mentality/.

Colmers, J. 2011. "The Once and Future Challenges of Implementing Health Reform." *The Commonwealth Fund.* Published November 14. www.commonwealthfund.org/Blog/2011/ Nov/Once-and-Future-Challenges-of-Implementing-Health-Reform.aspx.

Cooper, R. 2000. "Leadership Development Program: Knowledge-Intensive Growth at DuPont." *Wharton Leadership Digest*. Accessed September 28, 2012. http://leadership.wharton.upenn .edu/digest/07-00.shtml.

Corporate Leadership Council. 2005. *Realizing the Full Potential of Rising Talent*. Vol. I of *A Quantitative Analysis of the Identification and Development of High-Potential Employees*. Washington, DC: Corporate Executive Board.

Covey, S. R. 1990. *The Seven Habits of Highly Effective People*. New York: Free Press.

Dister, L. 2009. "CMO or VPMA—Is There a Difference?" *The Physician Executive* 35 (3): 12–16.

Drucker, P. 1973. *Management: Tasks, Responsibilities, Practices*. New York: Harper and Row.

Dye, C. F., and A. N. Garman. 2006. *Exceptional Leadership: 16 Critical Competencies for Healthcare Leaders*. Chicago: Health Administration Press.

Elliott, V. S. 2011. "Companies Express Confidence in Physician-Led ACOs." *American Medical News*. Published October 18. www.ama-assn.org/amednews/2011/10/17/bisd1018.htm.

Fields, R. 2011. "6 Issues Facing Hospital CEOs in 2011 and Beyond." *Becker's Hospital Review*. Published March 14. www.beckershospitalreview.com/hospital-executive-moves/6-issues-facing-hospital-ceos-in-2011-and-beyond.html.

Freudenheim, M. 2011. "Adjusting, More M.D.'s Add M.B.A." *New York Times*. Published September 5. www.nytimes.com/2011/09/06/business/doctors-discover-the-benefits-of-business-school.html?pagewanted=all&_r=0.

Gamble, M. 2012. "5 Hospital and Health System CEOs: What 'Top Performance' Looks Like to Me." *Becker's Hospital Review*. Published February 15. www.beckershospitalreview .com/hospital-management-administration/5-hospital-and-health-system-ceos-what-qtop-performanceq-looks-like-to-me.html.

———. 2011. "The Unhappy Physician: Why Hospitals Need to Take Morale Seriously." *Becker's Hospital Review*. Published December 5. www.beckershospitalreview.com/hospital-physician-relationships/the-unhappy-physician-why-hospitals-need-to-take-morale-seriously. html.

General Electric. 2012. "Leadership and Learning." Accessed September 28. www.ge.com/ company/culture/leadership_learning.html.

Goleman, D. 2000. "Leadership That Gets Results." *Harvard Business Review* March–April: 82–83.

Gulf South Quality Network (GSQN). 2011. "East Jefferson General Hospital Announces Collaboration with GSQN." Published February 3. www.gsqn.org/gsqnetwork.

Hennagir, J. F. 2012. "Huron Consulting Group Releases Huron Healthcare Report Providing Top Hospital Executives' Perspectives on Industry Issues for 2012." *Huron Consulting Group*. Published January 24. http://ir.huronconsultinggroup.com/phoenix. zhtml?c=180006&p=irol-newsArticle_Print&ID=1651685&highlight=.

Hogan, J., R. Hogan, and R. B. Kaiser. 2011. "Managerial Derailment." In *American Psychological Association Handbook of Industrial and Organizational Psychology.* Washington, DC: American Psychological Association.

Horney, K. 1937. *The Neurotic Personality of Our Time.* New York: W.W. Norton & Co.

Hughes, R. A. 2005. "Can This Marriage Be Saved? Physician–Hospital Relationships: Arizona Health Futures Policy Primer." *Saint Luke's Health Initiatives.* Accessed October 16, 2012. http://slhi.org/pdfs/policy_primers/pp-2005-12.pdf.

Institute of Medicine (IOM). 2012. "Best Care at Lower Cost: The Path to Continuously Learning Health Care in America." Published September 6. www.iom.edu/Reports/2012/Best-Care-at-Lower-Cost-The-Path-to-Continuously-Learning-Health-Care-in-America.aspx.

———. 2006a. *Preventing Medication Errors: Quality Chasm Series.* Washington, DC: National Academies Press.

———. 2006b. *Rewarding Provider Performance: Aligning Incentives in Medicare.* Washington, DC: National Academies Press.

———. 2003a. *Priority Areas for National Action: Transforming Health Care Quality.* Washington, DC: National Academies Press.

———. 2003b. *Patient Safety: Achieving a New Standard for Care.* Washington, DC: National Academies Press.

———. 2001. *Crossing the Quality Chasm—A New Health System for the 21st Century.* Washington, DC: National Academies Press.

———. 1999. *To Err Is Human: Building a Safer Health System.* Washington, DC: National Academies Press.

The Joint Commission. 2009. *Leadership in Healthcare Organizations: A Guide to Joint Commission Leadership Standards.* Published November 19. www.jointcommission.org/assets/1/18/WP_Leadership_Standards.pdf.

———. 2008. "Behaviors That Undermine a Culture of Safety." Published July 9. www.jointcommission.org/assets/1/18/SEA_40.PDF.

Kaiser, R. B. 2009. *The Perils of Accentuating the Positive.* Tulsa, OK: Hogan Press.

Katz, R. L. 1995. "Skills of an Effective Administrator." *Harvard Business Review* 33 (1): 33–42.

Kaufman, N. 2012. Presentation to the ProMedica Board Retreat, October 7.

Keckley, P. 2012a. "Health Care Reform Memo: October 22, 2012." *Deloitte Center for Health Solutions.* www.deloitte.com/view/en_US/us/Insights/Browse-by-Content-Type/Newsletters/health-care-reform-memo/704c18880588a310VgnVCM1000003156f70aRCRD.htm?id=us_email_CHS_HCRM_102212.

———. 2012b. "Health Care Reform Memo: May 14, 2012." *Deloitte Center for Health Solutions.* www.deloitte.com/view/en_US/us/Insights/Browse-by-Content-Type/Newsletters/health-care-reform-memo/d35c723d88b47310VgnVCM3000001c56f00aRCRD.htm.

Kotter, J. P. 2001. "What Leaders Really Do." *Harvard Business Review.* Published December 1. http://hbr.org/2001/12/what-leaders-really-do/ar/1.

———. 1996. *Leading Change.* Boston: Harvard Business Review Press.

Lasagna, L. 1964. "Hippocratic Oath—Modern Version." University of California, San Diego. Accessed December 4, 2012. http://ethics.ucsd.edu/journal/2006/readings/Hippocratic_Oath_Modern_Version.pdf.

Lehigh Valley Health Network (LHVN). 2008. "Leadership Development." Published December 19. www.lvhn.org/Physician_Careers%7C887.

Liebhaber, A., and J. M. Grossman. 2007. "Physicians Moving to Mid-Sized, Single-Specialty Practices. Tracking Report No. 18." *Center for Studying Health System Change.* Published August 1. www.hschange.com/CONTENT/941/.

Lindberg, L., and D. Paller. 2008. "Reaching Out to Physicians." *Trustee.* Accessed January 1, 2012. www.trusteemag.com/trusteemag_app/jsp/articledisplay. jsp?dcrpath=TRUSTEEMAG/Article/data/10OCT2008/0810TRU_DEPT_QualityUpdate &domain=TRUSTEEMAG.

Lombardo, M., and R. Eichinger. 2002. *The Leadership Machine.* Minneapolis, MN: Lominger Limited.

Maruca, W. H. 2009. "JCAHO Requires 'Zero Tolerance' for Disruptive Doctors and Administrators." Published January 1. www.foxrothschild.com/newspubs/newspubsArticle. aspx?id=7816.

Mayo Clinic. 2012. "Physician Well-Being Program." Accessed October 17. http://mayoresearch .mayo.edu/mayo/research/physicianwellbeing/.

———. 2002. "Mayo Clinic Model of Care." Accessed August 31, 2012. www.mayo.edu/pmts/ mc4200-mc4299/mc4270.pdf.

McCall, M. 1998. *High Flyers: Developing the Next Generation of Leaders.* Boston: Harvard Business Review Press.

Menaker, R., and R. S. Bahn. 2008. "How Perceived Physician Leadership Behavior Affects Physician Satisfaction." *Mayo Clinic Proceedings* 83 (9): 983–88.

Merry, M. 1996. "Physician Leadership: The Time Is Now." *The Physician Executive* 22 (9): 4–9.

Morrissey, J. 2010. "Evaluating Hospital–Doc Relations." *Modern Physician.* Published November 8. www.modernphysician.com/article/20101108/MODERNPHYSICIAN/3110 89954#ixzz1iFYpbjIh.

Morton, B. 2011. "The Ongoing Dynamics Between Physicians and Hospital Administration." *Morehead Associates.* Published April 7. www.moreheadassociates.com/blog/posts/the-ongoing-dynamics-between-physicians-and-hospital-administration.

O'Connor, E. J., and C. M. Fiol. 2006. "Reclaiming Physician Power: Your Role as a Physician Executive." *The Physician Executive* 32 (6): 46–50.

Page, L. 2010. "Cleveland Clinic's COO Marc Harrison Discusses Physician Leadership, Increasing Use of Data and Role of Employed Physicians." *Becker's Hospital Review.* Published February 10. www.beckershospitalreview.com/news-analysis/cleveland-clinics-coo-marc-harrison-discusses-physician-leadership-increasing-use-of-data-and-role-of-employed-physicians.html.

Paller, D. A. 2005. "What the Doctor Ordered." *Gallup Business Journal.* Accessed September 13, 2012. http://gmj.gallup.com/content/18361/What-Doctor-Ordered.aspx.

Peter, L. J., and R. Hull. 1969. *The Peter Principle.* New York: William Morrow and Company.

Prime Education. 2007. "Changing the Public Perception of Doctors." *PRIME.* Published June 1. http://primeinc.org/casestudies/physician/study/506/Changing_the_Public_Perception_of_Doctors.

Redding, J. 2012. Personal correspondence with author, October 31.

Riley, G. J. 2004. "Understanding the Stresses and Strains of Being a Doctor." *The Medical Journal of Australia.* Accessed October 17, 2012. www.mja.com.au/journal/2004/181/7/understanding-stresses-and-strains-being-doctor.

Roman, C. 2011. "Simple Steps to Improve Relations with Physicians." *Hospitals & Health Networks.* Accessed July 2, 2012. www.hhnmag.com/hhnmag_app/jsp/articledisplay.jsp?dcrpath=HHNMAG/Article/data/03MAR2011/0311HHN_Coverstory&domain=HHNMAG.

Routson, J. 2011. "Should a Physician Have an MBA?" *HealtheCareers Network.* Published April 19. www.healthecareers.com/article/should-a-physician-have-an-mba/161627.

Sacks, L. B. 2010. "Clinical Integrations: The Foundation for Accountable Care." Presented at the University of Iowa College of Public Health, October 22. www.public-health.uiowa.edu/hmp/symposium/pdfs/10-Presentations/Sacks.pdf.

Sheinwold, A. n.d. Public Quotes. Accessed September 4, 2012. http://publicquotes.com/quote/42188/learn-all-you-can-from-the-mistakes-of-others.html.

Sloan, S., and R. Fralicx. 2011. "Is There a Leader in the House?" *Hospitals & Health Networks Daily.* Published August 11. www.hhnmag.com/hhnmag/HHNDaily/HHNDailyDisplay.dhtml?id=4680008273.

Smith, M. K. 2001. "Chris Argyris: Theories of Action, Double-Loop Learning and Organizational Learning." *Encyclopedia of Informal Education.* Accessed October 5, 2012. www.infed.org/thinkers/argyris.htm.

Solomon, R. J. 2004. "Physician Leadership: A Roadmap for Health-System Change." *Journal of Medical Practice Management* 20 (1): 36–40.

Temple University School of Medicine. 2012. "Medical Education: Integrated Curriculum." Accessed December 4. www.temple.edu/medicine/education/mdprograms/medical_education/curriculum_overview.htm.

Thomas, R. J. 2008. *Crucibles of Leadership: How to Learn from Experience to Become a Great Leader.* Boston: Harvard Business Press.

US Department of Justice and the Federal Trade Commission. 1996. "Statements of Antitrust Enforcement Policy in Health Care." Published August 1. www.justice.gov/atr/public/guidelines/0000.htm.

Virginia Mason Medical Center. 2001. "Physician Compact." www.virginiamason.org/workfiles/HR/PhysicianCompact.pdf.

Wachter, R. M. 2004. "Physician–Hospital Alignment: The Elusive Ingredient." *Commonwealth Fund.* Accessed March 1, 2012. www.commonwealthfund.org/usr_doc/Meyer_hopital_quality_commentary_wachter.pdf.

Webber, M. 1998. "Why and How Successful Leaders Get Derailed." *Leadership Letters.* Accessed May 23, 2012. www.leadershipletters.com/1998/07/07/why-and-how-successful-leaders-get-derailed-%E2%80%93-part-1/.

Weinstock, M. 2011. "The New Physician Leader." *Hospitals and Health News Daily.* Published July 21. www.hhnmag.com/hhnmag/HHNDaily/HHNDailyDisplay.dhtml?id=250008112.

Wells Fargo. 2012. "Leadership Pipeline Program—Wholesale Banking." Accessed September 28. www.wellsfargo.com/careers/mbas_undergrads/undergrads/programs/leadership.

Zasa, R. J. 2011. "Physician-Hospital Joint Ventures: Alignment of Physicians with Hospitals." *Becker's Hospital Review.* Published September 8. www.beckershospitalreview.com/hospital-physician-relationships/physician-hospital-joint-ventures-alignment-of-physicians-with-hospitals.html.

Zismer, D. K., and J. Brueggeman. 2010. "Examining the 'Dyad' as a Management Model in Integrated Health Systems." *The Physician Executive* 36 (1): 14–19.

Index

About the Authors

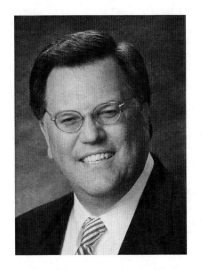

Carson F. Dye, MBA, FACHE, is an executive search consultant with Witt/Kieffer, which conducts chief executive officer, senior executive, and physician executive searches for a variety of healthcare organizations. His consulting experience includes leadership assessment, organizational design, and physician leadership development. He also conducts board retreats and provides counsel in executive employment contracts for a variety of client organizations. He is certified to work with the Hogan Assessment Systems tools for leadership assessment, selection, development, and executive coaching.

Dye worked for an international search firm before joining Witt/Kieffer, and before his search career served as the director of Findley Davies, Inc.'s Health Care Industry Consulting Division. Prior to his consulting career, he served 20 years as chief human resources officer at various organizations, including St. Vincent Medical Center, The Ohio State University Medical Center, Children's Hospital Medical Center, and Clermont Mercy Hospital.

Dye is a member of The Governance Institute Governance One Hundred and serves as a faculty member for The Governance Institute. He works as a special advisor and facilitator for The Healthcare Roundtable. In 1998, he was named as a physician leadership consultant expert on the Hoffmann–La Roche National Consultant Panel. He served on the adjunct faculty of the graduate program in management and health services policy at Ohio State University from 1985 to 2008 and currently teaches leadership for the University of Alabama at Birmingham in its executive master of science in health administration program.

Since 1989, Dye has taught several cluster programs for the American College of Healthcare Executives (ACHE) and frequently speaks for state and local hospital associations. He authored the 2001 James A. Hamilton ACHE Book of the Year winner, *Leadership in Healthcare: Values at the Top* (Health Administration Press 2000). He has written several books for Health Administration Press, including *Leadership in Healthcare: Essential Values and Skills* (2010), *The Healthcare C-Suite: Leadership Development at the Top* (2009), *Exceptional Leadership: 16 Critical Competencies for Healthcare Executives* (2006), *Winning the Talent War: Ensuring Effective Leadership in Healthcare* (2002), *Executive Excellence* (2000), and *Protocols for Health Care Executive Behavior* (1993). He has also written several professional journal articles on leadership and human resources.

Dye has had a lifelong interest in leadership and leadership assessment. He has studied how values drive leadership and affect change management. He is also a student of executive assessment and selection. Dye earned his BA from Marietta College and his MBA from Xavier University.

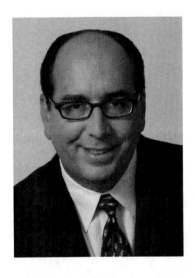

Jacque J. Sokolov, MD, is chairman and chief executive officer of SSB Solutions, Inc., a US-based healthcare management, development, and investment company. Following his formal training as an academic cardiologist, Dr. Sokolov has had the opportunity to serve as a board director, corporate officer, and advisor in multiple healthcare sectors. He currently serves as a director of Hospira; MedCath Corporation; the National Health Foundation; Phoenix Children's Hospital; Healthcare Community Development Group, LLC; and My Health Direct, Inc. He previously served as the vice president of healthcare for Southern California Edison Corporation; chairman of the board of directors for Coastal Physician Group, Inc.; chairman of the executive committee of the White House Health Project; and director of the American College of Medical Quality and the National Business Group on Health.

Dr. Sokolov received his BA in medicine from the University of Southern California (USC) and his MD from the USC School of Medicine. He completed his internal medicine residency at the Mayo Graduate School of Medicine and his fellowship in cardiovascular diseases at the University of Texas–Southwestern Medical School. He previously held and currently holds academic appointments and advisory board responsibilities in the schools of medicine, business, and public health at Harvard University; the Massachusetts Institute of Technology; the University of Pennsylvania; the University of California, Los Angeles; and USC.